CLINICAL SUPERVISION IN
Mental Health
Nursing

About the Author

Graham Sloan is a Clinical Specialist in Cognitive Psychotherapy and works in Consulting and Clinical Psychology Services, NHS Ayrshire and Arran. He completed his PhD in May 2004 studying with the School of Nursing, Midwifery and Community Health, Glasgow Caledonian University. He has had several papers relating to clinical supervision and cognitive and behavioural psychotherapy published in the recent nursing literature and has presented at international conferences. He provides clinical supervision to mental health nurses, cognitive and behavioural psychotherapists, clinical psychologists and psychiatrists and provides education on clinical supervision and CBP within the Trust. He is also employed as a Visiting Lecturer at Glasgow Caledonian University.

Foreword

At last, a research project on clinical supervision in nursing where we are left in no doubt as to what really happens in nursing supervision. With his debut book, Graham Sloan has produced both an enjoyable read, at once informative and rigorous, as well as an honest account of how supervision at least in one Mental Health site in Scotland has developed since its implementation. Gone are the usual wild claims and extravagant benefits made for the behalf of clinical supervision and in their place is a well-considered and cautiously executed study that allows the reader a view that is reliably absorbed in objective data. We know this because we are provided transcripts of actual accounts of supervision sessions recorded via audio-taping.

Sloan is not happy with the usual subjective reports of supervision that remain unquestioned; nor is he satisfied with the purported yet untested ideals found in the nursing literature – he wants to capture the essence of supervision first-hand and, unusually, in an empirical manner. To this end, his research questions propose gaining objective knowledge on the content of clinical supervision, how the interpersonal interactions between supervisee and supervisor influence this content, the impact of the organisation in which nurses work on the supervision process and the changes that are expected to occur in supervision. Uniquely to nursing supervision research, he uses an Illuminative Evaluative approach that focuses on the supervisory dyad couple and this method further enables him to encapsulate any modifications to the supervision process during its unfolding. After all, supervision is an ongoing dynamic process, and change is inherent to all dynamic processes.

To obtain his rich data base, Sloan collects multiple sources of information both from interviews and self-ratings of all participants and his own careful observations which he subjects to Burnard's (1991) thematic analysis and Heron's (1971) Six Category Intervention Analysis in a longitudinal study over 18 months. These methods provide him with an epistemically objective means of evaluating the interpersonal domain of subjective interactions, rather than merely relying on his own thoughts and biases. This is innovative and enormously important and has not been done before in nursing supervision. What Sloan has done here is to do elevate simple talking to the level of complex action – speech acts are acts like any other, and clearly have a reciprocal impact on both the listener and the speaker. Thus, he legitimises the 'talking approach' of clinical supervision, and for all nursing, not only for mental health nursing.

Rightly, Sloan argues that supervision is an educational innovation, and one that cannot be separated from the learning milieu or wider organisational context. It is highly interesting then, to note that, without exception, all supervisors in this study were on-line managers. The result is unsurprising. Most supervision discussions were underpinned by managerial concerns from the supervisor – a situation both contrary to the literature and contrary to what supervisor and manager participants themselves claimed. As promised by the expanding nursing literature, supervision is not particularly supervisee-led, and these supervisee-participants were not shy in disclosing to the researcher their dissatisfactions with supervision. Clearly, this is an unexpected benefit from the study in that the supervisees derived some benefit and even relief from discussing their experiences.

Sloan ensures, as much as possible, to 'keep himself out' of the participants' expectations of supervision; he has no need to 'influence' them to tell a researcher what he may want to hear. And he does this in the most sensitive manner – he informs all participants that he wants to know what is happening, and not what 'should' be happening. At every turn, he offers participants to review their statements or withdraw their audio-visual tapes recording their sessions. It is to his credit that, overall, the participants were as generous as they were, considering the sensitivity of their private thoughts and the knowledge that some of those thoughts would be published in a public world (although anonymously).

Sloan, too, is generous. He is overwhelmed with data, yet manages to offer the reader a coherently flowing account of his journey, selecting personal quotes that absorb our attention and make us want to think for ourselves. One cannot help but be left with the impression that his own work as a supervisor is highly sensitive and unambiguously on the side of the supervisee's self-discovery. He is disappointed that this does not happen more frequently either in the literature or in his study. Yet, with his unobtrusiveness he does not suggest what we should think – that is entirely left to us – the reader.

Sloan, sensibly, concludes that a complexity of factors influence how nurses engage with clinical supervision: the organisational culture and perception of supervision, who supervises, what training and ongoing support is offered to supervisors, what is hoped to be achieved, and for what outcome.

It also remains unanswered what is being 'supported' in supervision. The usual assumption is that nurses' wellbeing is supported in the light of the new therapeutic patient-centred nursing approach (Butterworth and Faugier, 1992; Savage, 1990), yet there is little evidence to substantiate this. No great in-depth discussions of the impact of patients on nurse's therapeutic work were uncovered in this study. Frustratingly so. But there are many insights to this study. My own favourite is this (though I am biased here): How clinical supervision is conceptualised by nursing scholars and practitioners will influence how supervision is implemented and developed. The repercussions are clear enough: much work still needs to be done on considering what nurses want or need from supervision rather than waxing lyrically about its untested benefits.

Further, it is not enough to just listen and accept to what people say they do, one must explore what actually happens in practice. There is no shame in this – all of us can misperceive our environment, or we can deceive ourselves, or simply be mistaken about what we think. I think this book deserves all the time and the effort required to study it, to savour it and to return to it for the insights that are glowing on many of its pages.

Tania Yegdich

Acknowledgements

I wish to record my thanks to all those who allowed me access to the research sites and would like to extend a special thank-you to the participants who gave their time and wisdom. Without their collaboration, this study could not have been undertaken. I hope that the experience has been of benefit to them.

I owe a great deal to my academic supervisors Professor Hazel Watson, Professor Jean McIntosh and Victor Henderson, an outstanding team of scholars, and feel privileged to have been guided by them. I am especially grateful for the careful direction, critical companionship and never-ending support offered to me by Professor Hazel Watson – thank you.

I am also grateful to the Director of Mental Health, the Research and Development Manager and the Director of Consulting and Clinical Psychology Services in the Trust where this study was conducted for supporting and providing the funding for the project. I am appreciative of the administrative assistance provided by Zoë Lawson, Anthea Moorhouse and Janette White.

I owe immense gratitude to my loving wife, Maureen, for all her selfless support, encouragement and understanding throughout the preparation of my PhD thesis and without whom I could not have done this – thank you.

I am grateful to the many friends and colleagues who have given their time, attention and support during the conduct of this research, particularly Dr Janice Harper, Dr Margaret Brown, Frank Coit and Beryl McFarlane.

Finally, I wish to acknowledge the inspiration and encouragement I was afforded during the early stages of my career by Rae Lind, George Findlay and John Ross, who, at the time, were nurse tutors at Dumfries and Galloway College of Nursing.

List of Figures

List of Tables

1 Introduction

BACKGROUND TO THE STUDY

INITIAL EXPERIENCES

I started my registered mental nurse (RMN) modular training in 1982. Clinical supervision (CS) was something I did not experience as a student. When I qualified in 1985, I worked for six months in an acute psychiatric admissions unit; again, CS was not available. It was when I took up the post of staff nurse (SN) in an adult psychotherapy day hospital that I was offered the first opportunity of CS. A psychoanalyst working in the unit provided CS; it was delivered in a group format, and all staff had to participate. There was a great deal of conflict among some members of the team and this animosity seeped into supervision. On reflection, in many ways supervision was used to contain team dynamics and provide an opportunity to explore staff relations. I do not recall client issues being discussed. I was uncertain of what I should be doing in CS, since being relatively new to the team I did not have any tensions with my colleagues.

Around the same period, the charge nurse (CN) started to provide individual CS to the nursing staff in the unit. At that time, CS had not stimulated much interest and there was a distinct lack of conceptual analysis and empirical research on CS and its relevance to nursing in the United Kingdom (UK). I did not receive any training in CS; nor was I given the option not to participate. As far as I can recall, the CN explained that CS would give me an opportunity to discuss my work with clients and anything that was of concern. Being a new member to the team, I had much enthusiasm for my work and wanted to fit in and create a good impression with my colleagues and line manager. At that time, I understood CS as a 'must do' activity and that it was provided by the CN.

I can recall talking about several clients, and in particular one gentleman who suffered from depression. He had been in and out of psychiatric hospitals most of his adult life and had been seen by numerous psychiatrists, psychotherapists, clinical psychologists and community psychiatric nurses. Throughout our contact, despite conveying a motivation for change, by asking for help, the client always appeared reluctant to engage in working on ideas that had emerged during sessions. In addition to feeling deskilled, I found myself irritated, confused and critical of his inability to take things forward.

What appeared to trigger my need to take these issues to CS was an awareness that my reactions and subsequent interactions with certain clients were not as helpful or enabling as I had intended. I was hopeful that through CS I would reach a better understanding of my clients, their needs and how I might contribute more effectively towards their recovery. Following my presentation of these clients, my supervisor would respond with supportive comments. I would hear him telling me how well I was doing and how impressed he was with my nursing care, compassion and persistence. Having my CN's approval was very important to me, and his comments were reassuring. From his perspective, I was doing OK. Nonetheless, I remained somewhat perplexed at my reactions when working with certain clients.

DEVELOPMENT

I have had many positive experiences with CS since my initial introduction. Its delivery has ranged between individual, group and triadic formats. Nursing staff who have undergone psychotherapy training have provided some of these experiences, and at other times CS has been provided by a psychiatrist, clinical psychologist or occupational therapist. I would argue that this consistent provision has assisted me in achieving a high standard of care. Intuitively, I would argue that the care I have provided to clients has benefited from my commitment to CS. Together with other professional development opportunities, consistent engagement with CS has progressed my professional competence. However, it has also had other significant benefits that are not as easily evidenced or appreciated.

As I alluded to earlier, engaging in a helping relationship is not always an easy or straightforward activity. Supervision has enabled me to tolerate my uncertainties when working with particular clients and helped me identify ways of working that have been positive for my clients, but which I have not always immediately acknowledged. It has assisted me in developing confidence in my provision of clients' care and has guided me towards appreciating unhelpful ways of working and supporting new ways of engaging with clients. In these contexts, in addition to CS being didactic and cognitive, it has facilitated the working-through of emotional material inextricably associated with my clinical work.

During the past 15 years, I have also provided CS to others. Initially, this was mainly to nursing colleagues but more recently has included consultant psychiatrists, clinical psychologists and nurses trained in cognitive and behavioural psychotherapy (CBP). The focus of the majority of this work has been facilitating the exploration of clinicians' therapeutic interactions with clients, their delivery of therapeutic interventions and reactions to this work.

CURRENT EXPERIENCES

Clinicians who approach me for CS usually have a desire to develop their therapy, and particularly the application of CBP. To assist in this process, I provide CS guided by Padesky's CBP supervision model (Padesky, 1996). I had been introduced to this framework 10 years ago and since then developed my understanding of its application. Attending training workshops on the framework has been beneficial. Supervision, guided by the CBP model, is similar to the therapy process in that it aims to be focused, structured, educational and collaborative. It also acknowledges that the practice of the supervisor and the supervisee (within and between supervision) will be influenced by their own core beliefs, underlying assumptions and automatic thoughts. In my role as clinical supervisor, I aim to help supervisees apply CBP to a high standard, develop their assessment, conceptualisation and treatment skills and, as advocated by Feasey (2002), explore their own reactions to the therapeutic process.

Personal experience suggests that this highly structured and clinically focused framework is a useful model for CS. The CBP supervision model remains loyal to the fundamental intention of CS – the development of therapeutic competence (Sloan *et al.*, 2000). Consequently, it is focused on the skills of therapy, their application by the supervisee, their impact on the therapeutic relationship and the alleviation of clients' psychological distress.

These recent experiences have reinforced my belief that the therapeutic relationship and the delivery of helpful interventions, particularly with mental health nursing colleagues, is an important focus for CS. Throughout their professional careers, mental health nurses are expected to engage with clients in an intentionally therapeutic manner and to ease clients' suffering by dealing with a heavy burden of emotional distress. Had I had the opportunity of CS during my early years as an RMN, which I receive currently, I might have gained a better understanding of the issues emanating from my relations with clients.

CLINICAL SUPERVISION IN NURSING

Despite having a presence in nursing since the 1920s (Burns, 1958), it is only in the comparatively recent past that an interest in CS in the UK has grown. It is well known that Florence Nightingale encouraged the supervision of junior nurses by more senior nurses to improve their practical skills (Abel-Smith, 1960). Nurse scholars from North America have written about the concept since the 1970s confining its use to psychiatric nursing, particularly for nurse therapists (Muecke, 1970; Termini and Hauser, 1973; Benfer, 1979; Critchley, 1987; Farkas-Cameron, 1995). According to Fowler (1996a), contemporary interest amongst UK nurses has been influenced by developments within the nursing profession, an increase in nurses' accountability, attempts to establish nursing as a profession and the recognition of the therapeutic focus of nursing.

In the UK, CS is now a frequently debated concept in nursing, as evidenced by the extensive literature on this topic in nursing journals. Many of the popular publications, for example *Nursing Times* and *Nursing Standard*, particularly during the latter part of the 1990s, regularly featured articles on CS. The scholarly journals *Journal of Psychiatric and Mental Health Nursing* and *Journal of Advanced Nursing* have provided a platform for critical debate from clinicians, educators and researchers. Furthermore, following the Butterworth and Faugier (1992) publication *Clinical Supervision and Mentorship in Nursing*, one of the first CS texts for nursing in the UK, several other books have been written (e.g. Bishop, 1998a; Bond and Holland, 1998; Power, 1999; Bassett, 2000; Driscoll, 2000a; van Ooijen, 2000; Cutcliffe *et al.*, 2001). There can be little doubt that a familiarity with CS is expanding within the nursing profession. Nonetheless, the differences between its representation as depicted by policy directives emanating from the Department of Health (Department of Health (DoH), 1993) and my own understanding stimulated a need for further critical appraisal.

DoH (1993) emphasises the development of CS as one of the key elements that enable nurses to maintain clinical competence, describing it as:

A formal process of professional support and learning which enables individual practitioners to develop knowledge and competence, assume responsibility for their own practice and enhance consumer protection and safety of care in complex situations. (DoH, 1993, p. 15)

In addition to acknowledging CS as a means by which nurses might receive support and learning, this description highlights the fact that CS is also expected to protect consumers from unsafe practices. I wondered if such a representation of CS might be guiding clinical supervisors towards closely monitoring their supervisees' practices.

OPPORTUNITY FOR RESEARCH

CS had been in existence for some time in the Mental Health Directorate (MHD) of the Primary Care Trust where I was employed. The clinical nurse manager (CNM) for the community mental health nursing service introduced CS during 1985. Prior to the director of nursing's (DN) initial attempts at the widespread implementation throughout the Trust in 1995, CS had not been available to hospital-based mental health nurses or general nurses and health visitors working in other clinical areas. The Trust's nurse advisor, whose role encompassed primary care nurses as well as mental health nurses, was responsible for the formation of a working group to consider the implementation of CS and to conduct an audit involving all qualified nurses. I was invited onto the working group but relinquished my membership when I commenced psychotherapy training.

The aims of the audit were to identify the current level of knowledge of CS in both hospital and community settings, highlight where CS was taking place and, if so, which models were in use, explore nurses' views on CS and their perceived advantages and disadvantages, and identify nurses' preferences on the grade, discipline and choice of clinical supervisors. Around the same time, members of the working group developed a discussion paper concerning CS that was made available to all nurses working within the Trust, a copy being held in every clinical area, ward and team.

Following this, four pilot sites were identified for the introduction of CS. Three of these sites were general nursing contexts and one was an acute admission unit within the MHD. However, this did not motivate other units within the hospital sector of the MHD to follow the initiative. At the commencement of the current study, despite CS being practised in the MHD of the Trust since 1985, no review or evaluation, formal or otherwise, had been conducted.

In 1996, I undertook a postgraduate diploma in cognitive and behavioural psychotherapy, during which I received CS. While I acknowledged the benefits of CS, I was aware that the focus during, and delivery of, CS was particularly valuable. On my return from the course, I began to provide CS to some nurses. I also engaged in much discussion with colleagues regarding the implementation of CS in other areas of the service. The views of those participating in CS were mixed, inconsistent and contradictory, a trend that appeared to resonate in much of the nursing literature.

In acknowledging the contrast between my own experiences of CS and those of colleagues and how it was being described in the nursing literature, I developed an interest in, and wanted to explore, what CS was being used for, how and who was providing it, how it was being practised and what sorts of issues would be discussed during CS. The time was right to undertake the present study.

Chapter 2 provides comprehensive coverage of the issues emanating from the expansive literature on CS and investigates the growing popularity of CS in nursing, benefit and outcome studies, characteristics of the clinical supervisor and interpersonal interactions during CS. Following this review, gaps in current knowledge were apparent. The research questions aimed at addressing these gaps and the methods required for this undertaking are described in Chapter 3. In Chapter 4, Heron's Six Category Intervention Analysis is described and an argument is presented for its use as an analytic framework, while Peplau's Theory of Interpersonal Relations is also discussed. Chapter 5 illustrates the study design and methods. Chapter 6 describes how this process was tested during a pilot study. Chapter 7 draws together the main findings and discussion. Finally, Chapter 8 sets out conclusions from the study and includes the major insights gained, the limitations of the study, its contribution to nursing and some recommendations.

I have been extremely privileged in having the opportunity to observe how others embrace CS. It is hoped that engaging in the research process has been of benefit to all participants and that the insights gained from this investigation are of benefit to those who participate in CS and its continuing development.

2 Literature Review

INTRODUCTION

The literature review presents a discussion of published work relating to CS that has been conducted over the past 30 years. An important aim of the literature review was to develop an appreciation of the current knowledge of CS in nursing in the UK. In particular, this chapter focuses on a critical appraisal of the empirical research. As a consequence of some aspects of CS being underdeveloped in nursing, the literature pertaining to other fields was also reviewed. The chapter begins with a review of the anecdotal accounts, expert opinion and position papers that have pervaded nursing literature during the past 15 years. Following an analysis and synthesis of current knowledge, a rationale for the investigation is proposed.

LITERATURE REVIEW STRATEGY

A comprehensive search of the current literature on CS was conducted. Literature was reviewed from a variety of sources. Keywords used to locate literature on health CD-ROMs (CINAHL, Medline, Psychlit and the British Nursing Index) included 'supervision', 'clinical supervision', 'support', 'stress', 'relationship', 'evaluation' and 'benefits'. This method of searching provided the foundation for the literature search. Reference lists in the literature sourced were also scrutinised for any potentially unlisted or inaccessible sources. Throughout the duration of the study, the researcher conducted periodic searches of these databases. A manual scrutiny of more recent journals was conducted to ensure that potential sources not yet listed in the computerised databases had not been overlooked. This search strategy was supplemented by networking with researchers and educators from the international community at conferences and workshops on CS. The Internet was also used to obtain useful resources related to the field of interest.

CLINICAL SUPERVISION: GROWING POPULARITY IN NURSING

The increasing popularity of CS in nursing has been highlighted by the plethora of articles featured in the leading nursing journals and the publication of related texts and policy statements. Some of this work has offered further clarification of the concept (Barber and Norman, 1987; Lyth, 2000). There have been reports of how it has been implemented in various nursing specialties (Duarri and Kendrick, 1999; Clough, 2001). Other articles give descriptions of specific CS models (Fowler, 1996b; Nicklin, 1997a; Rogers and Topping-Morris, 1997; Sloan *et al.*, 2000; van Ooijen, 2000). A minority of writers, namely Coombes (1997), Rogers (1998), Yegdich (1998, 1999a), Hyrkäs *et al.* (1999) and Gilbert (2001), offer constructive criticism of, and challenge to, ways in which CS is represented in nursing. Conversely, several authors, for example Faugier (1994), Bartle (2000) and Power (2000), purport a multitude of alleged benefits. However, before contemplating this work, reasons for the introduction of CS in the UK must be considered.

POLITICAL INFLUENCE

Although there has been a gradual growth in nursing's move towards CS, political support and recommendation by the profession itself and the UK Department of Health have given strong support to its potential influence. The Department of Health document (DoH, 1993) *A Vision for the Future* was one of the first to recommend that CS should be explored and developed. The practice of CS derived from the DoH (1993) definition, as clarified in Chapter 1, which required a formal, supportive process, the purpose of which was to enhance professional practice and care outcomes. Consequently, during CS all aspects of nursing practice were open to consideration. Moreover, this definition appeared to reinforce the United Kingdom Central Council for Nursing, Midwifery and Health Visiting's (UKCC, 1990) position on safe practice and the educational requirements of the nursing workforce: 'It [CS] is central to the process of learning and to the expansion of the scope of practice' (DoH, 1993, p. 15).

Following the Allitt Inquiry (Clothier *et al.*, 1994), the Chief Nursing Officer, Yvonne Moores, endorsed the quality assurance potential of CS. In a letter, which accompanied the distribution of a position paper on CS, she writes that:

> I have no doubt as to the value of clinical supervision and consider it to be fundamental to safeguard standards, the development of professional expertise and the delivery of care. (DoH, 1994a)

Support for CS in nursing appeared to result from the emphasis being placed on its ability to contribute to risk-management and an interpretation that it would ensure consumer protection. However, this assumed that those practitioners who were aware that they might be practising in a way that was risking patient safety would make such disclosures to their clinical supervisor. Similarly, it assumed that clinical supervisors, if able to recognise risk, would have the authority to deal with this in an appropriate and effective manner. Managerial responsibility in recognising negligent practices was never mentioned in these policy directives. It would appear that CS was being endorsed as a managerial resource.

In the following year, a review of mental health nursing (DoH, 1994b) emphasised the significance of 'high quality clinical supervision' for this speciality. In this report, CS is described as having many advantages (DoH, 1994b, p. 21):

- it places emphasis on clinical aspects of mental health nursing;
- it helps mental health nurses to assess training and research needs;
- it encourages the recognition and appreciation of individual clients and their social situation;
- it examines the multi-disciplinary contribution to comprehensive client care;
- it identifies and develops innovative practice;
- it creates an ethos that fosters staff retention and morale;
- it promotes vital links between research and clinical practice.

However, no description of 'high quality clinical supervision' was offered, nor was there any evidence supporting these reported 'advantages'.

Using six key statements, the UKCC (1996) delivered its much-anticipated position statement on CS, clarified the context within which it works and the principles that underpin its implementation. The Council argues that the potential impact on care and professional development for practitioners was enough to warrant investment. Nonetheless, the UKCC also suggests that potential benefits are not limited to patients, clients or practitioners: 'A more skilled, aware and articulate profession should contribute effectively to organisational objectives' (UKCC, 1996, p. 2).

In more recent years, following the introduction of clinical governance, Butterworth and Woods (1999, p. 2) remark: 'Participating in clinical supervision in an active way is a clear demonstration of an individual exercising their responsibility under clinical governance.'

Thus, the practitioner's responsibility for safeguarding high standards of care and continually improving the quality of their care, important issues for clinical governance, can be realised through CS (Cole, 2002; McSherry et al., 2002).

Such policy statements, by emphasising a quality agenda, raised the profile of CS. Consequently, this fuelled the expectations of nurse scholars, managers and clinicians. Not surprisingly, CS has been implemented into a broad range of clinical settings in various formats and guided by an assortment of frameworks.

FORMATS AND FRAMEWORKS

The UKCC's endorsement suggests that CS has something to offer nurses regardless of the clinical environment within which they work. Reports of how it has been introduced to district nursing, health visiting, mental health nursing, elderly mental health services, intensive-care nursing, a day-surgery unit, a haematology nursing development unit, theatre nursing, occupational health nursing and practice nursing have been published (Waterworth *et al.*, 1997; Landucci, 1998; Wright *et al.*, 1998; Bassett, 1999; Styles and Gibson, 1999; Ashmore and Carver, 2000; Clough, 2001; McFeely and Cutcliffe, 2001; Dixon and Bramwell, 2001; Smith, 2001; Spence *et al.*, 2002; Billington *et al.*, 2005). Descriptions of its implementation into these nursing contexts reveal how CS can be delivered in a variety of formats.

While Winstanley and White (2003) recommend that CS should take place either monthly or bi-monthly and, at the least, last for an hour, Adams (1991) reports supervisees receiving an hour of CS every three months. Individual CS is probably the most common mode of delivery in nursing in the UK (Kohner, 1994; Jones and Bennett, 1998; Duarri and Kendrick, 1999). In this context, and in keeping with UKCC (1996) recommendations, the clinical supervisor is often a nurse. It is frequently the case that the supervisor is also the supervisee's line manager (Swain, 1995; Scanlon and Weir, 1997; Davidson, 1998; Gilmore, 1999; Sloan, 1999; Lyle, 1998a; Veeramah, 2002; Duncan-Grant, 2003). However, descriptions of group and triad formats have also been published (Feather and Bissell, 1979; Winship and Hardy, 1999; Price and Chalker, 2000; Sloan *et al.*, 2000). Although uncommon, there have been accounts of CS where the supervisor has not been a nurse (Power, 1999; Sloan *et al.*, 2000). While researchers in the Scandinavian countries have evaluated the provision of group supervision (Segesten, 1993; Palsson *et al.*, 1994, 1996; Hallberg, 1995; Begat *et al.*, 1997; Severinsson and Kamaker, 1999; Arvidsson *et al.*, 2001), there has been little intentional empirical evaluation of any particular format in the UK.

Consideration must also be given to the conceptual framework guiding the delivery of CS. There are few theoretical frameworks that specifically explain the processes of CS as adopted in nursing. However, several nurse scholars have suggested frameworks used by other professional groups to conceptualise the purposes and processes of CS, for example Driscoll (2000b) describes a supervisory framework based on solution-focused therapy (de Shazer, 1985). A small number of authors have developed their own theoretical template. Nicklin's (1997a) practice-centred model and Faugier's (1998) growth and support model, for example, describe the broad purposes of supervision, illustrate important supervisory qualities, clarify roles for both the clinical supervisor and supervisee and offer direction on where to focus attention. There is little guidance in the nursing literature on the significant stages of the supervisory process, that is developmental theories.

Proctor's (1987) model has gained increasing popularity in nursing and is probably the most frequently cited supervision model in the UK nursing press (e.g. Faugier and Butterworth, 1994; Jones, 1995a; Cutcliffe and Proctor, 1998; Bartle, 2000; Cottrell, 2001). Its use has been advocated for a range of nursing contexts, for example mental health nursing (Faugier, 1996; Cottrell, 2001), practice nursing (Styles and Gibson, 1999), occupational health nursing (Bainbridge *et al.*, 2001) and medical and surgical nursing specialties (Butterworth *et al.*, 1997; Bowles and Young, 1999).

When using this model, supervisors can focus on all or any one of three areas at any time. In nursing's adoption of this model, the **formative** function is concerned with skills development and increasing the supervisee's knowledge; the **normative** function concentrates on managerial issues, including the maintenance of professional standards, and the **restorative** function is focused on providing support in an attempt to alleviate the stress evoked by doing nursing work (Jones, 1996; Cutcliffe and Proctor, 1998). The model does not provide any guidance on how a clinical supervisor might interact when working from any of its three functions.

Fowler (1996c) argues that there is not one model of supervision which will suit the needs of all nursing contexts. Any attempt to impose one model at the expense of others may be imprudent and create further problems for clinicians as they grapple with CS. As suggested earlier, supervisors using Proctor's model when working from its restorative function have nothing on which to base their interactions. Consequently, they would have to consult the wider literature in order to identify supportive interventions. In a similar vein, Glover (2000) speculates that a supervision model used in midwifery will not be relevant to psychiatric nurses and a model adopted in psychiatric nursing may not be applicable to health visitors. Of more relevance is the specific purpose for which CS is being practised. Health visitors and mental health nurses, if engaging in CS to help them explore their relations with clients, may both equally benefit from a supervision model promoting this focus. It is nevertheless important that descriptions of other supervisory frameworks are available.

Johns and Butcher (1993), Chambers and Long (1995), Fowler (1996c), Cutcliffe and Epling (1997), Driscoll (2000a) and Sloan and Watson (2002) describe a model based on Heron's (1989) theoretical framework. Descriptions of the Six Category Intervention Analysis (Heron, 1989) in the context of nurses pursuing a counselling qualification (Cutcliffe and Epling, 1997; Chambers and Long, 1995), pursuing a degree (Chambers and Long, 1995), working in respite care (Johns and Butcher, 1993) and paediatric nursing (Devitt, 1998) have been published. This framework differs from that developed by Proctor (1987) in that it turns attention to the interpersonal processes of supervision. Heron's framework is discussed further in Chapter 4.

Another supervisory framework taken from psychotherapy and adapted for nursing is the CBP supervision model. Todd and Freshwater (1999), Sloan *et al.* (2000) and Sloan (2006) highlight the usefulness of this psychotherapy supervisory framework, first described by Padesky (1996) and Liese and Beck (1997), for nursing. While Todd and Freshwater (1999) illustrate the similarities between reflective practice and guided discovery, Sloan *et al.* (2000) clarify that, while it was devised to help develop the therapeutic competence of cognitive therapists, the approach's use in nursing contexts merits consideration. In a more recent publication, Sloan (2006) describes how the clinical supervisor can assist the supervisee in exploring how their beliefs can impact on the therapeutic relationship with clients and, if unhelpful, how they can be modified. The CBP supervisory framework, by addressing both the processes and content of supervision, highlights its essential purpose: the development of the supervisee's therapeutic competence.

This model differentiates between modes and foci (Padesky, 1996). A supervision mode is the means by which supervisee learning and discovery occurs, for example case discussion, reviewing audio-recordings of therapy sessions or the provision of relevant educational material. The focus can include the mastering of new therapeutic skills, conceptualising a client's problems, progressing the therapist's understanding of the client–therapist relationship and working through the therapist's emotional reactions to their clinical work. These modes and foci appear relevant for the practice of CS in nursing where clinical practice has a therapeutic intention, and it is recognised that knowledge and skills may develop as a result of practitioners reflecting on their interpersonal relations with clients.

Some scholars, in developing their own frameworks, offer examples of further alternatives. Faugier (1998), for example, describes a growth and support model in an attempt to provide some guidelines to the characteristics of the supervisory relationship. Faugier argues that the role of the supervisor is 'to facilitate growth and provide essential support to the practice of clinical excellence' (Faugier, 1998, p. 25). It is essentially a guide for supervisors regarding the attitudes they express during CS. While it provides a broad range of characteristics, it was neither developed from, nor has it been evaluated by, empirical research.

Nicklin (1997a) developed a framework that addresses the purposes of supervision, the supervision cycle and aspects of the interpersonal process. In Nicklin's practice-centred model, Proctor's (1987) normative, formative and restorative functions are substituted with managerial, educational and supportive classifications. Furthermore, he transfers stages of the nursing process into a supervision cycle. He also gives attention to the interpersonal process by borrowing from Egan's (1975) counselling taxonomy. Empirical research relating to this model is critically analysed later in this chapter.

Rogers and Topping-Morris (1997) describe a problem-focused model. Using this model, the clinical supervisor can focus on clinical issues the supervisee is finding problematic. They suggest that it can also be used to resolve problems within the supervisory relationship, improve ineffective care plans and develop the supervisee's understanding of clinical issues for which they have no experience. Problem-orientated CS is described as a collaborative process through which problem-solving strategies facilitate the identification of solutions to the clinical problems recognised by the supervisee. While a strength of this model is that it is focused on the supervisee's clinical work, its emphasis on problems and ineffective care plans may undermine confidence. Furthermore, it appears to rely on the supervisee's ability to recognise clinical problems and that, once recognised, these would be shared during CS.

However, while there has been a gradual increase in the CS models described in the nursing press, Rogers (1999) suggests their uptake in specific nursing contexts is limited. Similarly, the research investigating the frameworks described by Nicklin (1997a), Rogers and Topping-Morris (1997), Faugier (1998) and Sloan et al. (2000) is scarce. Evaluating the effectiveness of Proctor's three-function interactive model has received attention in research conducted by Butterworth et al. (1997), Teasdale et al. (1998) and Malin (2000), which is reviewed later in this chapter.

Nonetheless, regardless of which framework has been adopted, CS is considered to have far-reaching benefits and potential outcomes. A great deal has been written about the expectations nurses have for CS, and a plethora of anecdotal accounts is depicted in the literature. These benefits have, according to Jones (1995a), become a mythologised element of supervisory practice.

CLINICAL SUPERVISION IDEALISED

By introducing formalised CS, anecdotal accounts and expert opinion suggest that nursing staff will develop their clinical competence and knowledge base (Chambers and Long, 1995; Nicklin, 1995; Porter, 1997), feel supported (Benfer, 1979; Cutcliffe and Epling, 1997; Wilkin, 1999), experience less stress, burnout and sickness absence (Firth, 1986; Wilkin, 1988; Faugier, 1994; Brocklehurst, 1998), develop personally (Butterworth and Faugier, 1992; Chambers and Long, 1995), be less inclined to leave nursing (Bishop, 1994), have an increase in self-confidence (Cutcliffe and Epling, 1997), feel less isolated (Cook, 1996), preserve or enhance their moral sensitivity in their work (de Raeve, 1998) and nursing practice will be better informed by nursing theory (Lowry, 1998). There has also been speculation that patient care will be improved (Bishop, 1994; Timpson, 1996; Goorapah, 1997). Furthermore, it has been claimed that health service organisations will also benefit by a reduction in the number of complaints to the health service (Farrington, 1995; Nicklin, 1995; Goorapah, 1997), standard setting and audit (Gorzanski, 1997), having a further risk-management tool (Tingle, 1995; Herron, 2000) and the promotion of the clinical-governance agenda (Butterworth and Woods, 1999; McSherry et al., 2002).

It is important to consider such expectations since in an indirect way they imply the ways in which practitioners must engage in CS. If improvement in clinical competence and knowledge were considered an appropriate benefit from participating in CS, discussion between supervisor and supervisee on clinical skills and associated knowledge would be expected. It is difficult to establish the origins of this plethora of expectations with any certainty. Perhaps expectations, which focus on the supportive nature of CS, derive from an early article written by Wilkin (1988), 'Someone to watch over me'. Wilkin highlights the loneliness and isolation when working as a community psychiatric nurse and stresses his need for CS:

> I soon began to feel vulnerable and isolated. There were times, especially after difficult sessions with clients, when I found myself sitting behind the wheel of my car feeling shell-shocked and wishing I could discuss my feelings with someone. (Wilkin, 1988, p. 33)

DoH (1993) supports the idea of CS: 'Nurses and health visitors require support in the development of their practice. One way of providing support is through the process of clinical supervision' (p. 15).

However, Faugier and Butterworth (1994), in describing Proctor's (1987) supervision model and Faugier's growth and support model, view 'support' as encompassing psychological support for nurses in order to alleviate the stress experienced by nurses. They explain:

> The 'restorative' or supportive function is a way of responding to the way in which nurses, engaged in intimate interactions with clients by the very nature of their work, necessarily allow themselves to be affected by the pain, distress, and disability of the clients. (Faugier and Butterworth, 1994, p. 17)

The Royal College of Nursing (RCN, 1999) along with several others, for example Coleman and Rafferty (1995), Fowler (1996c), Wray et al. (1998), Wilkin (1999) and Rafferty (2000), appear to endorse the use of CS to alleviate nurses' upset. Fowler (1996c) recommends cathartic interventions to assist with work-related distress, such as failure to get promotion, during CS. Coleman and Rafferty (1995) report that some practitioners had discussed personal problems and personal life events during CS. CS as a stress-relieving resource for nurses has been incorporated into the empirical evaluation of several investigations in the UK.

These claims, however, introduce a rather contentious issue. It has been suggested that there is an absence of supporting evidence for the alleged benefits of CS (Lyle, 1998b; Gallinagh and Campbell, 1999; Teasdale, 2000). There is a dearth of published research evidence to reinforce the claims that CS prevents nurses from leaving the profession, promotes clinical governance, reduces the number of complaints in the health service, is effective in risk-management or allows patients to notice a difference in their care, for example. Conversely, researchers in the UK claim that CS is an effective means

analysed using the Statistical Package for the Social Sciences, but the absence of detail concerning the statistical tests in Nicklin's report makes it impossible to judge the appropriateness of such analysis and casts doubt on his conclusions. Conversely, qualitative data from focus group interviews suggested respondents were satisfied with the opportunities to discuss and resolve stressful issues arising in the workplace.

This study attempted to incorporate methods of ensuring clinical supervisors adhered to the research protocol. The protocol required that the experimental wards complied with either a monthly or two-monthly regime of supervision. Non-compliance with the protocol was common with the volunteers and conscripts; respondents engaged in supervision on approximately one-half of the prescribed occasions. The majority of respondents in this study engaged in individual CS infrequently, on average once every two and a half months (Nicklin, 1997b). Consequently, the number of sessions reported was significantly fewer than what had been detailed in the research protocol. Failure to adhere to the research protocol by the conscripts is perhaps understandable. Conscripts may have engaged in the study without their full commitment, which raises concerns about the ethical implications of the study. Similar to Butterworth et al.'s (1997) study, there were no quality-control checks concerning the independent variable during the project to ensure supervisors were working within the **restorative** component.

The focus-group method is considered valuable in obtaining qualitative data (Basch, 1987; Kitzinger, 1995; McFeely and Cutcliffe, 2001). However, the validity of the data gained by Nicklin (1997b) must be challenged. In this study, the researcher was also responsible for the provision of supervision-skills training and facilitating the focus groups. In this context, it may have been difficult for participants to express negative opinions. Further, supervisors and supervisees were members of the focus groups; thus, there was a probability that neither group would express their full experience (Nyamathi and Shuler, 1990). Ideally, researcher and provider of supervisory roles should be separate in a quasi-experimental evaluation.

Sickness-absence days and the Maslach Burnout Inventory were also used by Dunn (1998) to evaluate Proctor's (1987) restorative function. At the time of her audit, 63 nurses working in various clinical settings throughout the Trust were receiving CS. The audit included five wards engaged in implementing CS and two control wards. Data were collected for six months prior to the introduction of supervision and for a six-month period following its introduction. Dunn (1998) highlights an increase in emotional exhaustion in both experimental and control wards, though the change seen in the experimental ward was slight. Dunn (1998) also notes a reduction in the sickness and absence records in the experimental wards. Importantly, it is highlighted that these changes cannot be regarded as the result of CS alone (Dunn, 1998). The lack of description of the wards used for both the intervention and control is an important omission. If experimental and control wards varied in speciality, staff resource, complexity of patient condition and length of patient stay, comparing results would not be appropriate.

A strength common to the research conducted by Butterworth *et al.* (1997), Nicklin (1997b) and Dunn (1998) is the use of a particular supervision model. As noted earlier, Proctor's (1987) model has been frequently described in the nursing literature. Returning to the original text clarifies her thesis:

> Both (*supervisor and supervisee*) carry some degree of responsibility for the development of the student or worker (the formative task). Both carry some share of the responsibility for the ongoing monitoring and evaluating of the student or worker and at certain times – at the end of a course or the point of promotion, for instance – either may carry responsibility for assessment (the normative task). Each carries a share of the responsibility for ensuring that the student or worker is adequately refreshed and re-creative (the restorative task). (Proctor, 1987, p. 24)

Since the model attempts to offer support (restorative function), it would appear that nurse scholars and researchers have assumed it would have the capability to reduce levels of stress, burnout and other aspects of psychological distress as experienced by supervisees. Findings from empirical research do not support this hypothesis, however (Gilmore, 1999). In addition to the relative inexperience of supervisors and the brief duration of the intervention, the influence of Proctor's model on the non-significant results requires discussion. The framework or model guiding the CS would appear to be an important aspect of the intervention. Thus, it is probable that Proctor's model and how it influenced participants' practice of CS had some bearing on the results of the research conducted by Butterworth *et al.* (1997), Nicklin (1997b) and Dunn (1998).

Proctor's model contains no description of those interventions that can be regarded as requisite for the pursuit of each of its functions; what supervisor–supervisee transactions might be considered appropriate when working in the 'restorative' domain? During the research projects conducted by Butterworth *et al.* (1997), Nicklin (1997b) and Dunn (1998), clinical supervisors may therefore have experienced difficulty when functioning within the restorative component of the model. Despite these studies having a quasi-experimental design, there does not appear to have been any effort made in standardising the intervention. Similarly, no checks were made to ensure clinical supervisors were continuing to use Proctor's model. Therefore, doubt can be cast with regards to precisely what it was these researchers were investigating. Ultimately, these researchers would be unable to conclude if it was the 'restorative' component that was responsible for any changes demonstrated. Further research focusing on supervisor behaviour when working with particular components of this model is necessary.

Teasdale *et al.* (1998) evaluate the CS that nurses were receiving in the Trent region of England. The authors hypothesise that nurses who received CS would report lower levels of burnout and feel more supported than nurses who did not. Information was collected from nurses (n = 211) who worked in both general hospital and community settings using a survey design that incorporated a critical incident questionnaire, the Maslach Burnout Inventory, the Nursing in Context Questionnaire and a background information questionnaire. Results were compared for two groups, those receiving CS and those receiving only their usual levels of informal support not involving CS.

Qualitative data generated from the critical incident forms were subjected to analysis, which followed the qualitative approach described by Glaser and Strauss (1967). The Maslach Burnout Inventory was analysed using a Chi-square test. Teasdale *et al.* (1998) state that they classified the sample as high-, low- and medium-risk groups such that the use of the Chi-square test would be appropriate. This afforded Teasdale *et al.* (1998) the opportunity to compare their results with Butterworth *et al.* (1997). However, in addition, they used the Mann–Whitney U statistic to investigate levels of burnout in the two groups. This resulted in a more robust analysis than that of Butterworth *et al.* (1997). Scores from the Nursing in Context Questionnaire were summed for each component factor before applying tests of significance. A *t*-test followed by multi-variate regression analysis was used. These methods appear to be appropriate to the data and purpose of analysis.

In Teasdale *et al.*'s (1998) investigation, data from the Maslach Burnout Inventory did not detect any protective effects against burnout, confirming the results of Butterworth *et al.* (1997), Nicklin (1997b) and Dunn (1998). Teasdale *et al.* (1998) conclude that CS does not appear to offer any protection against burnout, at least not among nurses with overall levels of burnout below the norms for the Maslach Burnout Inventory. It is possible that the duration of the intervention, that is participants receiving CS over a 12- to 18-month period, contributed to its failure in offering any protection against burnout.

The Nursing in Context Questionnaire is a relatively new measure developed by Brocklehurst, one of the research team. This measure comprises 18 attitude statements divided into three factors, measuring the extent to which nurses (i) perceive their managers as listening and supportive, (ii) cope with their work and workplace and (iii) successfully access support at work (Teasdale *et al.*, 2001). It was identified that the receipt of CS may be associated with higher levels of perceived support, particularly for hospital-based nurses of lower grades and receiving supervision from line managers.

This is a notable finding and suggests that the ways in which nurses engage with CS is influenced by their clinical grade and length of experience. Perhaps inexperienced nurses value CS more than experienced staff. Another important factor, but one overlooked by previous researchers, is concerned with the clinical grade of the clinical supervisor. Teasdale *et al.* (1998) identified that when nurses had a choice of clinical supervisor they chose a colleague; when supervisors were allocated, it was mainly G-grade managers and above who were taking on this role. A valuable focus of future research would be nurses and their clinical supervisors on particular clinical grades. The supervisory experiences of E-grade SNs being supervised by G-grade CNs, for example, require investigation.

Interestingly, nurses who engaged in CS also used informal supports for immediate support and advice, and there appear to be no difference in the type of incident and the outcome discussed in CS or informal support channels. Consequently, Teasdale *et al.* (1998) highlight the importance of maintaining a range of both formal and informal support for nurses, rather than opting exclusively for CS. These researchers also underline the difficulty in separating CS from other support mechanisms. Qualitative approaches, as an alternative to quasi-experimental and survey-type designs, may clarify these practices. The influence of organisational factors on how nurses engage with CS needs attention.

KNOWLEDGE DEVELOPMENT AND SKILLS ACQUISITION

In a recent document (UKCC, 2001), there is an acknowledgement of the potential for CS to reinforce lifelong learning for nurses. In the document, it is stated: 'Clinical supervision can help you to develop your skills and knowledge throughout your career . . . it is an integral part of your lifelong learning' (UKCC, 2001, p. 6).

Previously, in a National Health Service Management Executive document CS was described as:

> A formal process of professional support and learning which enables individual practitioners to develop knowledge and competence, assume responsibility for their own practice and enhance consumer protection and the safety of care in complex clinical situations. It is central to the process of learning and to the expansion of the scope of practice. (DoH, 1993, p. 15)

Similar aspirations are detailed in the United Kingdom Central Council for Nursing, Midwifery and Health Visiting's (UKCC, 1996, p. 2) position statement on CS: 'Clinical supervision assists practitioners to develop skills, knowledge and professional values throughout their careers.' The anecdotal evidence found in the nursing press began to receive some support from empirical work. Proctor's (1987) model has been a common feature in the studies conducted in the UK. Butterworth *et al.* (1997), Dunn (1998) and Malin (2000) investigated the formative component of this model. However, since this work concentrated on only one particular perspective, it does have limitations.

Butterworth *et al.*'s (1997) study incorporated the use of individual in-depth interviews (n = 34) to identify self-reported outcomes of CS. Fifty topics were collapsed into two categories: personal and organisational. Among the 45 personal outcomes were those changes that were practice-related. Rather than highlight changes in knowledge or skills acquisition, participants reported development in their self-confidence, the support from peers, a sense of taking responsibility for their practice, being more honest, relaxed, enthusiastic and less competitive. Nevertheless, the qualitative data collected from the interviewing process by providing essential insights into participants' experiences illuminated advantages of undertaking further qualitative studies of CS.

Several nurses who were participants in Butterworth *et al.*'s (1997) multi-site evaluation of CS were also involved in a more recent study (Hadfield, 2000). A semi-structured interview was designed to investigate particular situations, specific events and CS in the context of paediatric nursing practice. Within the interview schedule were three vignettes, which were developed by the researcher from Proctor's (1987) assertion that formative, restorative and normative elements are necessary in CS. Each vignette incorporated a principle that Hadfield (2000) thought requisite for effective CS, that is the mutuality of the supervisor–supervisee relationship, the interpersonal relationship and the predicament arising out of professional versus personal pressures. The vignettes, according to Hadfield (2000), enabled her to access participants' understanding of CS, their experience of it and their ideas about its continued utility.

Following data analysis, Hadfield (2000) asserts that patient care could be improved. Ten participants reported that CS had a positive effect on their clinical practice. Four were able to give specific examples, which were arranged into three categories: clinical events, interpersonal and practice difficulties and professional development. The following example illustrates changes in a participant's clinical work:

> Another participant talked about the tragic event of a child she was nursing who in fact died, and how CS helped her to talk about her practice in relation to the child and family, focusing on her communication and empathy. She firmly believes that she gave an improved quality of care, developed effective relationships with all concerned, paid more attention to detail and felt more committed. Although the child died she felt that she had provided good quality care. (Hadfield, 2000, p. 32)

Dunn (1998) identifies more-precise changes in participants' skill, knowledge and attitudinal development. A section of a semi-structured questionnaire asked supervisees to report whether or not their skill, knowledge and attitude to their work had changed as a result of clinical supervision and, if so, to give an example.

Respondents reported changes in both practice and knowledge. Changes to clinical practice included reviewing the patient hand-over, standard setting, using a behavioural analysis tool, addressing the spiritual needs of patients, patient-protection issues and serving patients their meals. Respondents also noted changes to their approach to work; interpersonal relationships were perceived to be more assertive and confident, for example. Changes in knowledge included being able to deal with aggression, reflect on practice, participate in team-building strategies and improved communication skills.

Malin's (2000) investigation of the effectiveness of Proctor's (1987) model focused on a specific specialty: a learning-disabilities service. In 1996, a group of 15–20 nurses and other care professionals working in three community homes and one community multi-professional team serving adults with a learning disability undertook a course on CS. During this, they were encouraged to adopt Proctor's supervision model and requested to participate in a pilot project. The Trust commissioned a small-scale evaluation to examine how the process of CS had been accepted, the gains achieved and what lessons had been learned. Malin (2000) set out to examine how CS was being interpreted, how it had been operating, its benefits to supervisees and the contribution of supervisors.

The method chosen was two-staged. First, observation and a critical incident form were used; second, a semi-structured staff interview schedule was designed. The researcher observed supervision sessions within three of the units on a total of five occasions and managed to secure three untaped individual supervision sessions and the taping of two group sessions. A fourth unit was not prepared to have their supervision sessions observed but agreed to complete critical incident forms covering the purpose and outcome of individual sessions. In total, 18 critical incident forms were completed by three trained and three untrained staff over a four-month period. Following this, an interview schedule was designed, circulated among unit staff for comment and amended accordingly. Interviews were conducted with 11 members of staff, seven registered nurses employed in community settings and four members of a multi-professional community learning-disabilities team: community nurse, social worker, psychologist and physiotherapist. All interviews were audio-recorded, content analysed and summarised to look for key themes.

Supervisees reported that CS had helped them improve teamwork relations and to reflect on the care they provided. Moreover, Malin (2000) attempted to uncover clinical supervisors' contributions to these changes. The researcher's primary intentions of observing supervision were to develop a suitable interview schedule. His requests to observe individual sessions were rejected. However, he was given access to group sessions and these were audio-recorded. As a result of this period of observation, Malin (2000) formulated the question: 'What type of skills based on your own experiences do you feel you employ as a supervisor (for example types of intervention: confronting/facilitator)?' Supervisors felt comfortable to impart knowledge. Conversely, they experienced unease when their delivery of CS merged with management agendas, for example disciplinary matters. This may have been because they acknowledged the tensions resulting from CS being provided by a manager. This is similar to what supervisees experience when CS and managerial supervisory boundaries merge (Butterworth *et al.*, 1997; Brooker and White, 1997; Cutcliffe, 2000a; Kelly *et al.*, 2001). The UK nursing literature highlights considerable support for the management-led model for the delivery of supervision. It is common for supervisory arrangements to be hierarchical, for example H-grade supervising G-grade supervising E-grade. However, its influence on how participants ultimately engage with CS and the relationship between managerial and supervisory roles requires further exploration.

Malin (2000) makes an important contribution to the field by attempting to capture the range of skills used by a clinical supervisor during supervisory discussions. In order to progress the field, further investigation of the clinical supervisor's contribution is necessary. Malin (2000) uses a series of focused questions, which may have restricted participants to describing either confronting or facilitator interactions. An inquiry into supervisors' interactions may be more effectively explored using explorative questioning.

Of significance is the fact that Malin (2000) was refused access to individual CS sessions in one unit, implying a reluctance of some participants in having sessions observed. The researcher's presence may have had detrimental consequences, stopped supervisees from discussing certain issues and stifled supervisors' delivery of interventions. His presence and its effect when observing individual and group sessions in the other three units are not discussed. Furthermore, observation of only a small number of supervision sessions was conducted in order to develop an interview schedule. Observation of supervision could be incorporated for the purpose of developing a comprehensive understanding of the supervisor's interactions. However, alternative methods to direct observation, and observation over a prolonged period, may be required.

Critical incident forms were incorporated when Teasdale *et al.* (1998) investigated the impact CS had on patient care. Both supervised and unsupervised nurses (n = 211) returned 156 completed critical incident forms. The nurses were asked to describe clinical events that they had discussed with their clinical supervisor or with a member of their informal support network. Respondents' accounts relate what they did in their clinical practice as a result of CS or informal support.

The critical incidents were mostly patient-focused and included concerns over how to respond to any deterioration in the condition of patients, how to deal with aggressive or violent behaviour, how to manage pain control or other medication issues and dealing with complaints. From the examples given, Teasdale *et al.* (1998) clarify the impact of CS on clinical practice. Future research could develop the use of critical incidents by requesting participants to complete a critical incident journal over an extended period of time. Moreover, research participants could be asked to describe events that they feel are related to what they have discussed during CS, thus linking changes in clinical practice to supervisory discussions.

The reliance on self-report data from the perspective of only the supervisees, however, must be cautioned as potentially diminishing the trustworthiness of data. Data could be gathered from both the clinical supervisor and supervisee – the supervision pair. Furthermore, a triangulation of methods could assist the collection of a comprehensive data set; individual interviews and critical incident journals could be incorporated. Initially, researchers wrote of triangulation as though it were merely the use of multiple methods for the sole purpose of attaining confirmation (Denzin, 1970). However, more recently this view has been extended to incorporate the purpose of 'completeness', which is particularly important for qualitative researchers. Completeness is concerned with using different methods within one study and is expected to contribute 'an additional piece of the puzzle' (Knafl and Breitmayer, 1991, p. 230).

With the exception of Malin's (2000) study, researchers have investigated knowledge and skills acquisition from CS with nurses working in various specialties, for example district nursing, health visiting and school nursing (e.g. Butterworth et al., 1997; Dunn, 1998; Hadfield, 2000). Self-report data indicate that these groups of nurses can describe changes in their knowledge and skills as a result of engaging in CS. Conversely, mental health nurses working in acute psychiatry were unable to identify what skills they attained from supervision, or in what areas CS improved clinical outcomes. According to Jones and Bennett (1998, p. 22), this suggests that a considerable amount of resources are being applied to a phenomenon that in relation to patient care has 'no clear attainable benefits'. However, this finding may have highlighted a limitation of self-report data and mental health nurses' inability to articulate changes.

CONFIRMATION OF THE NURSE'S ROLE

Confirmation of what nurses do as an effect of CS is mainly confined to research conducted in the Scandinavian countries. In this body of work, supervision has been delivered in a group format by a supervisor with extensive CS training (Palsson et al., 1994; Begat et al., 1997; Arvidsson et al., 2000). In all studies, the source of confirmation has been derived from both verbal and nonverbal interactions amongst other group members. Findings from Hadfield's (2000) study, in addition to reporting that CS had a positive effect on clinical practice, also suggest that it helps to confirm nurses' work. One respondent explained that CS gave her the opportunity to explore difficult cases that facilitated a deeper reflection on her work. Through exploration and focused reflection, this respondent's practices were confirmed.

SUMMARY OF BENEFIT AND OUTCOME STUDIES

At the commencement of this chapter, the idealised benefits and expectations, as depicted in the mass of nursing literature pertaining to CS, were clarified. Evaluation research has provided minimal support for many of these claims. Currently, there is no empirical evidence to substantiate the claim that CS reduces the number of nurses leaving the profession, reduces the number of complaints, facilitates standard setting, bridges the theory–practice gap, enhances nurses' moral sensitivity to their work or prevents nurses from feeling isolated. Findings which claim that CS develops nurses' clinical competence and knowledge base, improves the quality of patient care, supports nurses and improves their emotional well-being are inconclusive. Continuing to search for specific, predetermined and considerable outcomes from this single process may prevent other, less substantial, changes being noticed.

It may be necessary to consider how other variables influence the practice of CS. Minimal attention has been afforded to the particular characteristics of the supervisee, their length of experience and qualifications, their motivation and capacity to be self-reflective. Furthermore, aspects of the clinical environment and their influence on CS have been overlooked. Future research may be required to take cognisance of the clinical environment, speciality, patient complexity, throughput and other workload issues.

In the process of reviewing the research measuring the effectiveness of CS on nurses' well-being and knowledge and skills acquisition, a significant oversight is apparent. The investigations in this review have given minimal attention to aspects of the supervisory process, for example supervisor style or the adherence to a particular supervisory framework. This creates some difficulty when clinicians are faced with implementing a study's recommendations. Similarly, researchers have a difficulty in replicating the intervention since they have nothing on which to model their provision of CS.

Butterworth *et al.* (1997), Nicklin (1997b) and Dunn (1998) do progress the field in nursing; all studies set out to investigate Proctor's (1987) supervision model. However, none of this work discusses the significance of the supervisory relationship; there has been an absence of focus on the interactions between clinical supervisor and supervisee. The essence of the supervisory relationship has not been captured. Consequently, the interpersonal interactions that take place within the supervisory relationship which contribute to knowledge development and confirmation of the nurse's role remain enigmatic. Uncertainty continues to permeate the nursing literature concerning those aspects of the interactions between clinical supervisor and supervisee that have been potent in assisting with any change. Furthermore, the necessary features of 'high-quality clinical supervision' in the context of mental health nursing (DoH, 1994a) require investigation.

Yet, in nursing, the supervisory relationship is considered an important aspect of CS (Trainor, 1978; Platt-Koch, 1986; Faugier, 1994; Bond and Holland, 1998; Chambers and Cutcliffe, 2001; Jones, 2001a, 2001b). Indeed, Faugier and Butterworth (1994) provide guidelines on 13 supervisor qualities they feel characterise a positive supervisory relationship. In the descriptions of their own CS models, Nicklin (1997a) and Rogers and Topping-Morris (1997) allude to the interpersonal relationship underpinning CS. Bond and Holland (1998) assert that the quality of the supervisory relationship has an important influence on the overall effectiveness of CS. The multiplicity of definitions and their contents circulating in the nursing literature reinforce this argument. In addition to implying particular benefits for the recipients of supervision, a significant relationship demanding a level of interpersonal competence is uncovered. For example, the Community Psychiatric Nursing Association (CPNA, 1985, p. 4) refers to a 'dynamic, interpersonally focused experience'; Barber and Norman (1987, p. 56) highlight 'an interpersonal process'; Butterworth and Faugier (1992, p. 12) describe 'an exchange'.

There is little evidence in the research literature of any attention afforded to this specific aspect of CS in nursing. Nonetheless, a small quantity of work attempts to clarify the helpful characteristics of the clinical supervisor.

CHARACTERISTICS OF THE CLINICAL SUPERVISOR

CHARACTERISTICS OF A GOOD SUPERVISOR: A NURSING PERSPECTIVE

Findings from research emanating from North America and Scandinavian countries, for example the work of Pesut and Williams (1990), Severinsson (1995) and Severinsson and Hallberg (1996), because of the ways in which their particular healthcare systems are organised, the peculiarities of nursing practice and a different understanding and utilisation of CS, may not be entirely relevant to nursing in the UK. Unlike the research conducted in North America and Scandinavian countries, which focuses on the perceptions of the clinical supervisor, research in the UK investigating the desirable characteristics of a clinical supervisor focuses on the supervisee's perspective.

Using a combination of quantitative and qualitative methods, Fowler (1995) was the first nurse researcher in the UK to investigate desirable characteristics from the supervisee's perspective. The aim of the first and second stages of the study was to collect qualitative data regarding the characteristics of a good supervisor. Stage three used the qualitative data to inform the development of a questionnaire for distribution to a larger sample in stage four.

During stage one, a short questionnaire was given to 30 post-registration students who were doing a 24-week full-time English National Board (ENB) clinical award course. The clinical award course consists of 40% taught theory and 60% clinical practice. During clinical placements, students are required to have a supervisor. The questionnaire focused on this individual and the relationship between student and supervisor. Only six of the 30 students (20%) opted into the study.

For the second stage, the researcher conducted a focus-group discussion involving the six participants. Students were encouraged to identify characteristics of a good supervisor and record these on a flip chart. Themes were identified and prioritised: values you as an individual, values your own role and shows it, demonstrates effort and puts themselves out and relevant knowledge and ability to show it. A questionnaire based on data from stage two and the literature was developed (stage three). The questionnaire was divided into four sections. Section A dealt with general biographical details and sections B, C and D addressed the characteristics of the supervisor. This was distributed to 38 post-registration students on a 24-week ENB specialist award course and seven post-registration students on a higher award course.

The majority of the students confirmed all of the qualities and areas identified in the first two stages of the study as being important. In summary, good supervisors are knowledgeable and can communicate this knowledge in an understandable way, they discuss their previous knowledge and experience with the student and, in addition to giving criticism, they comment on good practice.

Participants in this study identified teaching and supervisory skills as separate characteristics. That is, for these supervisees, it was not enough that their supervisor could create supportive relationships and have the relevant clinical and theoretical knowledge; their supervisor also had to have a certain degree of teaching competency. This characteristic may have been prioritised with this particular sample since they were students undertaking further college-based study. In this context, Fowler's (1995) research could be considered as being concerned with preceptorship rather than CS. Furthermore, the applicability of the study's results to other supervisees not necessarily engaged in supervision while undertaking further education is questionable. The small sample size also limits the generalisability of the results. Nevertheless, focusing on supervisees' perceptions rather than supervisors' views represents a major shift from earlier work conducted in North America and Scandinavian countries.

Sloan (1999) developed this work further by conducting a descriptive investigation of the characteristics of a good clinical supervisor with SNs working in a mental health setting. A different clinical supervisor supervised each SN. The study was based on the first two stages of Fowler's (1995) study. From a convenience sample of eight nurses completing the questionnaire, six participated in a focus group. The focus group's discussion was audio-recorded, transcribed verbatim and subsequently analysed using Burnard's (1991) thematic content analysis. The nominal group technique was used to prioritise the characteristics identified during the focus group's discussion.

The ability to form supportive relationships, having relevant knowledge and clinical skills, expressing a commitment to providing CS and having good listening skills were perceived as important characteristics. Supervisees viewed their supervisor as a role model, someone who they felt inspired them, whom they looked up to and had a high regard for their clinical practice and knowledge base. The perceptions of SNs, working in a mental health specialty and receiving individual CS, of supervisor characteristics are consistent with Fowler's (1995) findings. Nonetheless, the short questionnaire may have constrained participants' initial expression of their supervisory experience. Semi-structured interviews may have been more suitable. Furthermore, no generalisations can be made from findings from such a small convenience sample.

Fowler (1995) and Sloan (1999) offer no description of the CS framework guiding what the research participants received. It is therefore difficult to place the characteristics identified in the context of a particular supervisory framework. Additionally, it makes comparisons with previous and future research an arduous task. Nonetheless, their work provides some insights into supervisees' perceptions of the desirable characteristics of CS.

In the absence of nursing research focusing on the interpersonal interactions during CS and only a small number of studies investigating good characteristics of the clinical supervisor, a review of related fields in nursing was necessary. The literature pertaining to preceptorship and mentorship was consulted. Similar to the CS literature, it became apparent that there was a lack of any empirical investigation into the interactions occurring between either mentor and mentee or preceptor and preceptee. It was therefore necessary to search the literature relating to other professional groups, namely counselling, psychotherapy and clinical psychology. This search was focused on identifying empirical work that investigated effective characteristics of CS and aspects of the supervisor–supervisee relationship.

COUNSELLING, PSYCHOLOGY AND PSYCHOTHERAPY

Research focusing on characteristics of the clinical supervisor is widespread in the counselling, psychology and psychotherapy disciplines. Most of this research has been carried out in North America. While findings from this body of literature, because of the peculiarities of their clinical practice and understanding and utilisation of CS, may not be entirely relevant to nursing in the UK, it was necessary to consider the approaches and methodologies of these studies.

The supervisee perspective has been emphasised and accorded significant attention. The research conducted by Worthington and Roehlke (1979), which focuses on both the supervisor and supervisee perspectives, is the exception. The dominant research approach in this body of work has been the survey using questionnaires pertaining to counselling and psychotherapy (Nelson, 1978; Heppner and Roehlke, 1984; Worthington, 1984; Allan et al., 1986; Rabinowitz et al., 1986; Carifio and Hess, 1987).

Effective supervisor characteristics appear to be stable across the disciplines. These include allowing the supervisee to directly observe their supervisor's clinical practice, for the supervisors to directly observe or review either a video- or audio-recording of supervisees' therapy sessions (Nelson, 1978; Worthington and Roehlke, 1979), having an interest in supervision (Nelson, 1978), utilising role-play during supervision to demonstrate interventions, providing relevant literature, encouraging the use of newly acquired skills

(Worthington and Roehlke, 1979; Heppner and Roehlke, 1984), giving guidance with treatment planning, advice and direction with interventions (Worthington, 1984; Rabinowitz *et al.*, 1986) and having relevant experience as a therapist and theoretical or technical knowledge (Nelson, 1978). The ability to provide a supportive relationship was common to all investigations.

In contrast to the survey design, Worthen and McNeill's (1996) phenomenological investigation of 'good' supervisory events used interviews to explore the supervisory experiences of counselling psychologists (n = 8) undergoing psychotherapy training. This study identifies similar findings to the surveys conducted by Heppner and Roehlke (1984), Allan *et al.* (1986), and Carifio and Hess (1987). All participants described their supervisor as conveying an attitude that manifested empathy, a non-judgemental stance towards them, a sense of validation or affirmation and the encouragement to explore and experiment. Participants believed that their supervisors helped to normalise their 'struggle'. This was often facilitated by personal self-disclosure from their supervisor. In this study, self-disclosure from the supervisor played a significant role in helping less experienced supervisees to reduce negative attributions of their behaviour and decrease anxiety by allowing them to normalise and tacitly re-label 'mistakes' as learning experiences. All participants referred to the quality of the supervisory relationship as crucial and pivotal.

There has been a plethora of supervision research conducted in the psychotherapy, psychology and counselling professions. A proportion of this work has attempted to gain some understanding of the characteristics that are considered 'good' and contribute towards supervision being a rewarding, satisfactory and worthwhile experience. The survey has been a popular research approach adopted for the investigation of effective characteristics of the supervisor. However, one difficulty with this method is selective response rates. Only participants who feel particularly strongly about a topic may respond. Respondents may misunderstand the questions or feel they cannot express their views satisfactorily. This may have occurred in Rabinowitz *et al.*'s (1986) study since respondents were required to complete a two-part supervision checklist, which consisted of a mixture of fundamental concepts from various contrasting theoretical orientations. The 12-item critical incident checklist attempts to identify issues raised during CS, which may, in fact, never occur, owing to the particular psychotherapy model being adopted. Moreover, this work has incorporated questionnaires peculiar to the fields of psychotherapy and counselling. Consequently, questionnaires such as the Psychotherapy Supervision Inventory (Nelson, 1978) and the Supervisor Behaviour Questionnaire (Worthington and Roehlke, 1979) were considered unsuitable for investigating this aspect of CS in nursing. However, the interview method has gained valuable insights into this aspect of the supervisor's contribution.

A number of researchers have turned their attentions from desirable characteristics towards the interpersonal interactions between the clinical supervisor and supervisee during CS sessions. Supervisees in these studies have been students undertaking additional counselling or psychotherapy training. The indirect observation of clinical supervisor and supervisee interactions has been a common method of data gathering, video-recording or audio-recording supervision sessions, for example. In the majority of studies, which were carried out in North America, the supervisor has been described as an experienced or excellent clinical supervisor (Goin and Kline, 1974; Holloway, 1982; Holloway and Wampold, 1983; Shanfield et al., 1993; Keller et al., 1996).

INTERPERSONAL INTERACTIONS DURING SUPERVISION

Goin and Kline (1974) claim that their work was the first of its kind in the field. The study was conducted at a psychiatric outpatient clinic and involved five clinical supervisors supervising second-year psychiatric residents. As part of the ongoing evaluation of the preparation of psychiatric residents, it was acknowledged that particular supervisors were consistently ranked 'outstanding'. The researchers video-recorded, via a one-way mirror, the supervision sessions of five 'outstanding' supervisors with their particular residents. Two supervisors were consistently rated as 'outstanding', the remaining three as good.

Each supervisor and their psychiatric resident had been meeting for supervision for approximately seven months before the recordings commenced. The sessions were video-recorded for three consecutive weeks. By the third session, participants reported the meetings to be quite like regular ones. The video-recording judged as most typical was analysed, one tape from each supervisory dyad (a total of five tapes). The tapes were first analysed, by a research psychologist and two psychiatrists experienced in therapy and teaching, to develop a checklist covering all of the subjects talked about by the supervisors. The checklist was not subjected to further validation. From this, it was apparent that the supervisors' comments fell into four general categories: statements focusing on remarks made by the patient, those that reflected the residents' needs, those concerning the supervisor and those giving information about technique, psychotherapy principles or general psychiatric knowledge. A table was designed with 16 types of statements covering all possible remarks.

Using this checklist, the researchers then analysed the supervisors' video-recording. Each remark a supervisor made was reviewed and a tick was placed on the checklist opposite the categories in which it belonged. Once each of the supervisors' comments was assigned to its appropriate category, a determination could be made of each supervisor's areas of emphasis. The next stage of analysis involved the supervisor and resident reviewing the video-recordings of supervision in the presence of one of the researchers. They were asked to stop the tape each time the supervisor made a comment they felt had been 'helpful'. These were then assigned to one or more of the 16 checklist categories.

Fifteen and twenty-one per cent of comments made by the two supervisors ranked as 'outstanding' were categorised as information-giving comments about psychotherapy technique. Conversely, only 2%, 5% and 9% of comments made by the three supervisors deemed 'good' fitted this category. For the 'outstanding' supervisors, over 50% of the helpful comments were defined by the residents as directed towards teaching about the techniques or principles of psychotherapy. For the other supervisors, no more than 33% of their comments fitted these categories. These findings are confirmed by the findings from the work of Nelson (1978), Worthington and Roehlke (1979) and Rabinowitz *et al.* (1986). Supervision is considered most effective, from the supervisee's perspective, when the supervisor provides guidance with treatment planning and advice and direction about interventions.

The work of Goin and Kline (1974) incorporates an innovative data-gathering method, the video-recording of supervision sessions. From this, they identified particular supervisor behaviours considered typical during their routine delivery of supervision. Despite supervision sessions being video-recorded, clinical supervisors reported that by the third recording their sessions were similar to 'routine' sessions, highlighting the brief time it took participants to feel comfortable with the recording equipment. This also illustrated the need to record sessions over a period of time, for example recording a session ad hoc or using data from only the first session may have captured supervision dissimilar from the 'routine'.

Holloway (1982) investigated the sequential patterns of verbal behaviour with five supervisors and their supervisees. Each supervisor was supervising four trainees. Supervision pairs were asked to audio-record sessions three, six and nine of their supervision. One of the trainees declined from having sessions audio-recorded. The total number of supervision sessions available for recording was 57; owing to machine malfunction or error, 14 sessions were inaudible. Thus, 43 audio-recordings were used in the analysis. However, only 20 minutes of each tape were rated for subsequent analysis.

Each 20-minute segment of the audio-recorded session was coded using a modified version of the Blumberg Interactional Analysis (BIA). The BIA is a system for coding supervisor–teacher interactions (Blumberg, 1970). It comprises 15 response categories: ten categories describe supervisor behaviour, four categories describe trainee behaviour and one category codes silence. The original 16 categories were collapsed to 11: five categories describe supervisor behaviour, four describe trainee behaviour, number ten codes silence and number 11 codes playing the tape of the trainee's counselling session. An independent rater trained in using the modified BIA and not acquainted with any of the participants coded all segments of data.

From these data, evidence for repetitive patterns of verbal behaviours between supervisor and trainee was confirmed. Of particular note, when supervisors used supportive communication, including reflection of feelings, direct praise and development of the trainee's ideas, they elicited the trainees' positive social emotional behaviour. When supervisors directly questioned opinions and suggestions from the trainees, they were faced with silence. Supportive communication kept trainees talking but did not help them to elaborate on their ideas. Evidence supporting the ways in which supervisors could encourage trainees to progress their skills acquisition was lacking. However, this may have been related to the use of only 20 minutes of the supervision session, particularly the ten- to 30-minute segment of a session. Perhaps supervisor behaviours relating to skills acquisition occurred at other points in a session.

Holloway justifies using the 20-minute segment. She wanted to avoid the social comments that usually occur at the beginning of a session and avoid variability in the length of scored periods due to the premature termination of some sessions (Holloway, 1982). It would have been beneficial if Holloway had piloted this approach; her assumptions concerning the beginning and end of sessions could have been tested. Indeed, 40 minutes of each supervision session were not analysed.

In a later study, Holloway and Wampold (1983) investigated the verbal patterns of behaviour in the supervision interview with staff supervisors (nine) and counselling trainees (30). Five supervisors had four trainees, three supervisors had three trainees and the remaining supervisor had one trainee (30 supervision pairs). Supervision pairs met weekly for a one-hour supervision session. An audio-recording of supervision sessions three, six and nine was requested. A total of 90 supervision sessions were recorded. Eleven of the audio-recordings were inaudible, resulting in a final data set of 79 recordings. Similar to a previous study (Holloway, 1982), the audio-recordings were coded using a modification of the BIA. However, in this study, two independent raters coded the complete hour of the supervision session rather than a 20-minute segment.

At the end of these sessions, both parties were asked to complete independently a satisfaction measure. The measures used, the Supervisor Personal Reaction Scale and the Trainee Personal Reaction Scale, were derived from the Therapist Personal Reaction Scale and the Client Personal Reaction Scale (Holloway and Wampold, 1983). Both measures have 32 items that are rated on a five-point Likert scale.

Findings from this investigation confirmed Holloway's (1982) previous results and, specifically, the use of repetitive messages during supervision. Clinical supervisors engaged in supportive communication, asking for information in response to trainee requests. However, Holloway and Wampold (1983) identify additional behaviours. They found supervisors being defensive or critical in response to the trainees' similar behaviour. Results from the satisfaction measures indicated that the trainees and supervisors devalued these behaviours. It is understandable that participants found being asked a question in response to their own questioning unsatisfactory. Similarly, it is easy to sympathise with participants' dislike for defensive and critical responses. However, with supportive qualities being acknowledged as a necessary 'good characteristic' (Heppner and Roehlke, 1984; Rabinowitz *et al.*, 1986), the finding that both supervisor and trainee devalued supportive communication is unusual.

Nonetheless, supervisors rated their own behaviour positively when they followed trainees' sharing of ideas with a request for further exploration and discovery. Similarly, trainees rated themselves positively when supervisors requested them to elaborate on their ideas. Perhaps trainees felt encouraged that their supervisor was interested enough to follow up on their ideas. However, supervisors devalued trainees' supportive responses and elaboration of their (the supervisors') ideas.

While Holloway and Wampold (1983) increased the segment of the audio-recordings for analysis from Holloway's (1982) study, their focus on only sessions three, six and nine of weekly supervision results in a snapshot perspective. While creating a larger, more cumbersome, database, the continuous indirect observation of supervisor–supervisee interactions over time would be useful in determining the stability of behaviours.

In a more recent investigation, a multi-disciplinary research team studied the process of CS in an accredited doctoral training programme (Keller *et al.*, 1996). An aspect of this research set out to answer the questions:

- What is the nature of supervision?
- What patterns of interaction can be identified in the process of supervision?

Participants included 11 supervisees, who were second-year students on a marriage and family therapy training programme, and four clinical supervisors, who each had over 15 years of supervisory experience. Twelve videotapes were subjected to analysis by observation, summarising, cross-checking, note-taking and summarising of themes. The research team subdivided into three teams of two and developed a consensual agreement about the themes of supervision and patterns of interaction. Participants were also interviewed. In relation to their question 'What is the nature of clinical supervision?', four themes emerged: 'imparting knowledge', 'self-understanding', 'hierarchy' and 'reciprocal hierarchy'.

Supervisors were able to impart their knowledge by several methods: the transmission of ideas, skills, techniques, wisdom, expertise, insight and modelling. Data from the interviews were supportive of these observations. Supervisees described the nature of supervision as: giving specific advice, helping the supervisee to clarify their conceptualisations about clients and making sure those conceptualisations fitted with the therapy model. However, some of these behaviours highlighted a supervisor's powerful hierarchical position, from which a 'hierarchy' theme was derived. The observers interpreted supervisor behaviours 'asking most of the questions', 'giving advice' and 'taking responsibility for the case' as hierarchical. Supervisees also had an ability to control the sessions; excessive talking, changing the subject and asking the supervisor personal questions gave them some hierarchical position during sessions.

Keller *et al.* (1996) suggest a four-stage process that depicts patterns of interaction in supervision. The researchers observed a 'nesting' stage where supervisor and supervisee would create a feeling of comfort by joint greetings, casual conversation and humour, which they label 'rapport-building'. The next stage, 'getting down to work', represented the engagement of supervisor and supervisee in the discussion of a clinical case. This finding confirms Holloway's (1982) assumption that there is a period of social greeting at the commencement of supervision. Moreover, Keller *et al.* (1996) highlight the importance of this phase in progressing to the next stages of the supervisory process. During the 'getting down to work' phase, supervisor behaviours were focused on the supervisee's involvement with the case; assessment, intervention options and rationale for interventions were explored. Interestingly, it was noted that, during the 'resolution of questions raised and options discussed' stage, occasionally the supervisee would ignore suggestions from the supervisor. The 'wrapping-up' stage was similar to the 'rapport-building' in that it was less formal than other aspects of the process and contained more chitchat.

The combination of the video-recordings and interviews appeared to develop the comprehensiveness of the data. Keller *et al.* (1996) gathered observational data from a small number of video-recordings to progress understanding of the process of a supervision session. Recording supervision sessions over a longer timeframe might facilitate a more detailed exploration of the processes of CS. Despite collecting observations of supervisory interactions using video-recordings, Keller *et al.* (1996) make little reference to the relevance of non-verbal and paralinguistic aspects of communication. The finer subtleties of interpersonal relationships, tone of voice, gaze, silences and proximity, in the context of CS, remain hidden.

Keller *et al.* (1996) did not return to participants for feedback on the analysis of behaviours observed. I would argue the importance of seeking participants' views on such analysis. Otherwise, misinterpretations and biases may prevail, particularly when researcher and supervisor roles are combined. This may have been problematic in Keller *et al.*'s (1996) research and may have threatened the trustworthiness of the analysis; some of the supervisors were also members of the research team and therefore knew what aspects of their supervision were being studied. Where interactions are being investigated, it would be more beneficial if participants were not privy to how their interactions were being investigated and analysed.

Goin and Kline (1974) and Keller *et al.* (1996) incorporate the use of video-recordings to explore interactions during supervision. Despite this, much of the data analysis related to the verbal interactions rather than the non-verbal behaviours normally observed using this type of media, raising the possibility that video-recording may have been unnecessary.

A proportion of the supervision research conducted in the psychotherapy and counselling professions has incorporated a specific framework for data analysis. Holloway (1982) and Holloway and Wampold (1983) use the BIA framework. The BIA has been used to analyse teaching and supervisory inter-actions. This framework, having a reasonable coverage of teaching categories, may be appropriate for the investigation of the supervision of trainees of psychotherapy and counselling. Nonetheless, its use in nursing research, investigating CS with qualified practitioners, may be limiting. CS appears to be adopted for reasons other than teaching when utilised in nursing contexts. Furthermore, nursing practice exceeds a counselling role. Alternative frameworks, which could be used for the analysis of interpersonal interactions within the context of nursing and the engagement of CS, require exploration.

DISCUSSION

In UK studies evaluating the effectiveness of CS, the supervisory intervention, as a new innovation to the ward or clinical area under investigation, usually lasted for a 12- to 18-month period. Yet, the expectations of what could be achieved were considerable. A particular expectation purported in the popular press in nursing, which has received considerable interest within the research community, is that of stress-relief for the supervisee. The empirical work supporting the effectiveness of CS as a stress-relieving resource can be challenged. When using the Maslach Burnout Inventory, GHQ-28 and sickness-absence rates to measure its effectiveness, findings are inconclusive. The expectation that CS will reduce stress, burnout and sickness absence is perhaps optimistic. Conversely, the changes resulting from CS as a supportive enterprise may not be sufficient to be revealed by standardised measures, particularly when baseline measures are mild or show no 'caseness'. It may be that in the quest to demonstrate the stress-relieving qualities of CS other potential changes may have been overlooked.

Research that has investigated the effectiveness of CS as a stress-relieving mechanism in the UK has been criticised. Gallinagh and Campbell (1999, p. 53) argue that 'confusion exists with regards to its purpose and effects'. The use of health-related questionnaires and particular statements made by nurse scholars might augment the viewpoint that nursing's understanding of CS extends beyond its traditional teaching focus, as illustrated in Chapter 1. In nursing, as suggested earlier, it would appear that CS incorporates a supportive purpose for the supervisee, which is regarded as having therapeutic qualities. This notion has been reinforced when comparisons have been made between the uses of CS in nursing and counselling. For example, Hadfield (2000, p. 31) writes: 'The relationship that is labelled clinical supervision could be understood at this point as not unlike a counselling relationship.'

It has been argued that the notion of CS being a vehicle for the provision of therapy only illuminates a conceptual misunderstanding. Yegdich (1999a) emphasises the misconception of CS in nursing, particularly with reference to the assumption that CS can enhance both professional development and personal growth. She stresses that nurses should refine the professional self during CS, not the personal self: 'talking about patients and one's therapeutic work, in preference to oneself and one's personal issues, is the cornerstone of supervision' (Yegdich, 1999a, p. 1272). By combining the two processes of personal and professional growth into one, Yegdich (1999a, p. 1273) suggests that 'a poor representation of both therapy and supervision is yielded'. North American nurse scholars have advocated a similar stance (e.g. Termini and Hauser, 1973; Gregg et al., 1976; Platt-Koch, 1986; Minot and Adamski, 1989; Farkas-Cameron, 1995).

It could be argued that an additional benefit of professional development is some positive shift in one's personal development, for example developing practice in using solution-focused therapy and observing the benefits of the approach in a client may contribute to an increase in self-confidence at work. An increase in self-confidence in the work context may enhance self-confidence in other areas. Nonetheless, as highlighted previously, it is the assumption that CS should target the personal growth of the supervisee that pervades the UK nursing literature. Consequently, this endorsement, as supported by the UKCC (1996) and prominent nurse scholars, may be widespread in the nursing community.

Evident from previous research in nursing was the lack of focus on clinical supervisors' interventions during a supervision session or their consequences. Indeed, despite the supervisory relationship being highlighted as **the** important component, it has received minimal attention from the nursing community. There is good reason to address this by examining what actually happens during supervision, what supervisors and supervisees actually do, what changes in the supervisee's practice are discussed and what, if any, changes occur in patient outcome. These questions may only be answered by focusing more on the CS sessions themselves, and by using multiple sources to provide data about the supervisory experience and longitudinal designs to examine the interpersonal processes over time.

A quasi-experimental approach has been commonly adopted to investigate the introduction of CS to nursing contexts. On average, the CS has lasted for between 12 and 18 months. It has been highlighted that in some NHS Trusts CS has been in place for several years (Bishop, 1998b). There is a need to investigate these experiences of supervision. Furthermore, the organisational context within which CS is practised and how this affects its nature and processes has not been given adequate attention. Consequently, the ward or team climate within which nurses work, the nature of nursing work, how supervision is understood and the supervisory relationship are contexts relating to CS that require investigation. Greater attention to what issues are taken to CS and how this is processed may provide opportunities to observe changes as reported by the supervisee. However, the illumination of multiple perspectives is necessary. To date, the experiences and perceptions of only clinical supervisors, supervisees or both have been investigated. If consideration is afforded to some of the contexts that affect the provision of CS, the opinions and perceptions of other stakeholders should be explored.

In light of findings from previous research conducted in the UK, particularly the work of Teasdale *et al.* (1998), it would be valuable to investigate CS as experienced by nurses working at specific clinical grades. Similarly, the provision of supervision from supervisors at specific clinical grades should be explored. This might provide information on how and in what ways particular grades influence how practitioners participate in CS.

Research conducted in the psychotherapy fields that has focused on supervisor–supervisee interactions during supervision illustrates the reciprocal nature of supervisory interactions. Supervisor behaviours provoke a reaction in the supervisee; supervisee response, in turn, determines subsequent behaviour from the supervisor. Future nursing research should turn attention towards the reciprocal interactions occurring during supervision between the clinical supervisor and the supervisee. By doing so, the ways in which CS facilitates the confirmation of nurses' work, particularly the clinical supervisor's interactions, may be illuminated.

CONCLUSION

This chapter presented a comprehensive review of the theoretical and empirical literature pertaining to CS in nursing in the UK. As a result of some aspects of this concept being underdeveloped, related fields both within and outwith nursing were considered. To develop this field of knowledge in nursing, it was argued that future research should turn attention to the supervisory relationship and its related processes. With this in mind, Chapter 3 presents the questions the current study set out to investigate.

3 Methodological Considerations

INTRODUCTION

Following a review of the theoretical and empirical literature, gaps in the current understanding of CS emerged. In particular, it was argued that research investigating aspects of the supervisory relationship and its influence on outcomes has been uncommon. In previous work, nurse researchers have tended to focus on aspects other than the interpersonal transactions between supervisor and supervisee. This chapter presents the general aim, research questions and objectives central to the current study. The relevant methodological considerations are then discussed. Thereafter, a rationale for the research approach and its methods is provided.

GENERAL AIM OF THE STUDY

To explore and describe the content of, processes within and changes resulting from the practice of CS by mental health nurses working in a National Health Service (NHS) Primary Care Trust.

RESEARCH QUESTIONS

Within this NHS Primary Care Trust:

1. What is the content of individual CS for mental health nurses?
2. How do the interactions between clinical supervisor and supervisee during supervision sessions influence its content?
3. How do the organisational factors of CS affect the supervisory process?
4. What changes are reported from this experience of individual CS?

OBJECTIVES OF THE STUDY

1. To identify the uses of individual CS made by mental health nurses working in an NHS Primary Care Trust.
2. To explore and describe supervisees' experiences of individual CS.
3. To describe how the organisational provision of CS influences the supervisory process.

4. To analyse the interactions between supervisor and supervisee during supervision.
5. To explore how these interactions influence the content of supervision.
6. To illuminate the changes resulting from supervision, as reported by participants.

CHOICE OF RESEARCH APPROACH

The present project was concerned with discovering the changes reported by mental health nurses engaging in CS. However, unlike previous nursing research in this field, the focus for the study also emphasised an exploration of the processes inherent with CS. Essentially, I wanted to uncover how the reciprocal interpersonal exchanges between supervisor and supervisee influenced what the recipient experienced from CS. This would involve paying close attention to interactions during supervision, examining what happens in supervision, what supervisors and supervisees actually do and what changes in the supervisee's practice are discussed. Consequently, this investigation required a research approach that would allow an exploration not only of its content and integral processes but also of the changes resulting from CS. These issues could only be addressed by focusing more on the CS sessions themselves, by using multiple sources of data concerning the supervisory experience and within a longitudinal design and by examining the changes reported by the supervisee over time. Similarly, it was necessary to explore these aspects during the routine delivery of CS as it occurred in its natural context.

The general aim and subsequent research questions place as much emphasis on processes as on changes (effects) and how these are achieved. It was therefore considered that the aim of the study would best be met by employing an evaluation approach which could acknowledge the complex interactive processes at work. Developmental evaluation, according to Øvretveit (1998), aims to describe the intervention and the people who use it in order to give an alternative perspective on the value of the intervention. Evaluations of this type are made when the item to be evaluated is difficult to specify, poorly defined, where there are mixed views on its format and purpose or when it is likely to change while the evaluation is being conducted. It has been suggested that there are many different types of developmental evaluation but all share certain features:

- local: done in one organisation but with the aim of producing general descriptions and knowledge that are useful elsewhere;
- no controls: no attempt to control the evaluated or to create experimental and control groups, but may compare case sites;
- non-experimental design: the evaluation is not designed as an experiment to treat a hypothesis;

- inductive: concepts and theories are built up inductively out of the data;
- a preference for qualitative techniques.
  (Øvretveit, 1998, p. 126)

Illuminative evaluation, developed by Parlett and Hamilton (1972), utilises a descriptive approach to evaluation. Illuminative evaluation represents a holistic approach which is responsive to the influences that occur in a given context. Accordingly, illuminative evaluation was adopted as the method for the current investigation.

ILLUMINATIVE EVALUATION

Illuminative evaluation is not a standard methods package but rather a general research strategy. Parlett and Hamilton (1976, p. 92) state: 'illuminative evaluation, like the innovations and learning environments that they study, come in diverse forms'. The approach emphasises the flexible selection of methods according to the participants and the opportunities that arise. The problem being investigated dictates the data-collection methods. Parlett and Hamilton (1976) propose that a triangulation strategy not only facilitates the viewing of a problem from a number of perspectives but also aids the confirmation of less definite findings. The use of multiple sources of evidence allows an investigator to address a range of historical, attitudinal and observational issues. Thus, any finding or conclusion in an illuminative-evaluation investigation is likely to be more comprehensive and convincing if it is based on several different sources of information. The triangulation principle was considered to be important for the current investigation. Previous evaluative research on CS in nursing has generally focused on one perspective, for example clinical supervisor or supervisee. A research approach using the collection of a variety of types of data from multiple sources was felt to be advantageous.

Illuminative evaluation was originally born from a dissatisfaction with traditional research approaches found in the evaluation of mainstream education programmes. Parlett and Hamilton (1972) suggest that conventional objective approaches to evaluation were inadequate for highlighting the complex problems of education (Melton and Zimmer, 1987). Instead, they developed a revelatory approach, which focuses on an innovation in its natural context. Illuminative evaluation follows an inductive process and is particularly appropriate when evaluation purposes require exploration that leads to description, understanding and decisions to effect improvements rather than prediction, formal hypothesis testing and measurement. Determining changes on outcome measures is not the goal (Shapiro *et al.*, 1983). Instead, the intended focus is on the performance that takes place in the natural context of the learning milieu with the aim of bringing the participants' experiences to light.

Central to understanding illuminative evaluation are two concepts, namely the instructional system and the learning milieu. Parlett and Hamilton (1972) argue that in traditional approaches to the evaluation of educational programmes there is a failure to recognise the 'catalogue' for what it is. The catalogue, or instructional system, is an idealised specification of a new programme and often contains grand objectives, a new syllabus and details of teaching techniques and equipment. The traditional researcher would build a study around innovations specified in this way and would administer tests most appropriate to evaluate the programme's objectives and determine if it had attained its performance criteria. Parlett and Hamilton (1972, p. 10) claim: 'this approach ignores the fact that an instructional system, when adopted, undergoes modifications that are rarely trivial'. In the practice setting or the learning milieu, grand objectives, as outlined in the instructional system, are commonly re-ordered, re-defined, abandoned or forgotten. While the concept of the instructional system has most relevance in educational contexts, its usefulness can be justified in a study of CS in clinical practice.

There is wide agreement that CS serves an educational purpose (Proctor, 1987; DoH, 1993; UKCC, 1996; Anderson and Dorsay, 1998; Chorley and Kitney, 2000; Kelly et al., 2001). A recent UKCC document states that 'clinical supervision can help you to develop your skills and knowledge throughout your career. It is an integral part of your lifelong learning' (UKCC, 2001, p. 6). CS could be considered as an educational innovation. Consequently, the 'instructional system' was understood as any organisational policy statements that set out guidance for the implementation of CS and educational descriptors of CS courses which practitioners had attended. Furthermore, the general themes evident in the wider CS literature pertaining to nursing were deemed relevant. The contribution this body of literature makes to the ways in which CS had been adopted cannot be overlooked.

Parlett and Hamilton (1972) argue that when an innovation ceases to be an abstract concept or plan, and becomes part of the teaching and learning in an organisation, it assumes a different form. This is clarified when they state:

> The theatre provides an analogy – to know whether a play works one has to look not only at the manuscript but also at the performance; that is, at the interpretation of the play by the director and actors. It is this that is registered by the audience and appraised by the critics. Similarly, it is not an instructional system as such, but its translation and enactment by teachers and students, that is of concern to the evaluator. (Parlett and Hamilton, 1976, p. 100)

Parlett and Hamilton (1976) put forward the notion that there is no play that is 'director-proof' and, equally, no innovation that is 'teacher-proof' or 'student-proof'. This scenario has similarities with how CS has been implemented in Trusts throughout the UK. According to Yegdich and Cushing (1998) and

Stevenson and Jackson (2000), the expectations of CS extend beyond its traditional and focused educational function. CS, as practised in other healthcare professions, was intended as an educational process aimed at progressing the supervisee's therapeutic competence (Loganbill *et al.*, 1982). This purpose has support in nursing (Platt-Koch, 1986; Farkas-Cameron, 1995; Anderson and Dorsay, 1998; Yegdich and Cushing, 1998). However, as highlighted in Chapter 2, in nursing, CS is also expected to deliver much more. Just as there may be no play that is director-proof or no educational innovation that is teacher-proof or student-proof, CS may not be practitioner-proof or researcher-proof.

The socio-psychological and material environment in which clinical supervisors and supervisees work represents a nexus of cultural, social, institutional and psychological variables. Parlett and Hamilton (1972) argue that acknowledging the diversity and complexity of the 'learning milieu' is an essential prerequisite for the serious study of educational programmes (innovation). They stress that innovations cannot be separated from the learning milieu or organisational context of which they become part. The introduction of CS to any healthcare setting is likely to precipitate a series of repercussions throughout the learning milieux within any organisation. Simultaneously, these consequences may affect CS itself, changing its form so that it no longer resembles its original representation (Yegdich and Cushing, 1998). According to recent government documents, it could be argued that any healthcare organisation could be considered a potential source for lifelong learning (DoH, 1999).

The 'learning milieu' and how it influences the utilisation of CS has been overlooked in previous nursing research adopting a quasi-experimental design. Furthermore, despite CS having a considerable history in some Trusts (Bishop, 1998b), there has been minimal empirical work which has explored the ways in which nurses engage with this resource in their natural settings. Nonetheless, researchers have commented on organisational factors, for example ward climate and its potential effect on CS (Hallberg and Norberg, 1993; Berg *et al.*, 1994; Dunn, 1998). Mental health nurses often find themselves working in particular service areas, for example an admission ward, day-care facilities, rehabilitation services or community mental health teams. Staff working within such areas recognise and identify with the 'team'. In each of these teams, a learning milieu consisting of particular ways of working, clinical priorities and team membership may contribute towards practitioners' experiences of CS. It was suggested in Chapter 2 that the future study of CS should acknowledge the diversity and complexity of the wider organisational context, that is the learning milieu. Parlett and Hamilton's (1976) consideration of the 'learning milieu' has relevance to question three of the present investigation: 'How do the organisational factors for clinical supervision affect the supervisory process?' Before considering possible data-gathering methods for an illuminative-evaluation study, a discussion on how it has been incorporated, particularly in nursing research, is necessary.

PREVIOUS ILLUMINATIVE-EVALUATION RESEARCH

Illuminative evaluation has its origins in the field of educational research. Since its inception, it has been used to investigate a range of educational activities, for example learning styles (Miles, 1981), curricula in mainstream education (Sharp, 1990; Burden, 1998), a management-training programme (Shapiro et al., 1983), the Open University (Melton and Zimmer, 1987), an agricultural-development project (Lee and Schute, 1991), social work evaluation (Gordon, 1991), a residential outdoor education centre (Robinson, 1991) and the health needs of ethnic minority groups in the UK (Hennings et al., 1996). Miles (1981) describes the 'instructional system' as an assemblage of diverse factors, including people, expectations, jargon and plans of the innovation. He explains: 'it is not a clear-cut set of skills and knowledge, but becomes melded with people and settings and actual attempts to make change' (Miles, 1981, p. 494).

Melton and Zimmer (1987) argue that illuminative evaluation facilitates the emergence of different perspectives. Shapiro et al. (1983) conclude that, rather than being product-focused, illuminative evaluation emphasises a focus on the processes integral to management training. Gordon (1991) argues that the precise measurement of intended outcomes is not the priority. Rather, illuminative evaluation allowed Gordon (1991) to explore what social workers were doing and how they could improve the ways in which they practised.

ILLUMINATIVE EVALUATION IN NURSING RESEARCH

Nurse researchers have adopted illuminative evaluation to investigate entire academic programmes (Chambers, 1988; Smith et al., 1995; Hamlin, 1996; Veitch et al., 1997), particular modules from various nursing courses (Crotty, 1990), educational approaches used in nurse education (Barber and Norman, 1989; Dewar and Walker, 1999) and aspects relating to the preparation of nurse teachers (Mhaolrunaigh and Clifford, 1998). This research has been conducted in nursing colleges mainly. Observation, interviews, questionnaires and documents have been a frequent method of data gathering in the majority of this research.

Smith et al. (1995) used interviews, observation and a questionnaire to collect data for an investigation of the health-promotion component of nursing, health visiting and midwifery curricula. A purposive sample of participants from five settings, which included lecturers, representatives from local health-promotion units, hospital and community staff and pre- and post-registration students, was used. A team of three researchers gathered data over five days per centre. However, the brief time used in Smith et al.'s (1995) study was deemed insufficient for this study. The current study required a similar duration as the work of Butterworth et al. (1997), Nicklin (1997b) and Dunn (1998) in order to achieve the objectives presented earlier. Moreover, it was felt that a prolonged engagement of 12- to 18-month duration would enhance the credibility and trustworthiness of the data.

Multiple perspectives were explored in a novel project, conducted by Dewar and Walker (1999), investigating work-based learning within a post-registration community health nursing degree programme. This project, one of the few exceptions in nursing, used illuminative evaluation to explore learning in the clinical environment as well as the academic setting. That is, the learning milieu included both educational and clinical contexts. Similar to the study conducted by Smith *et al.* (1995), Dewar and Walker (1999) collected data by various means, for example by questionnaire, observation and focus groups. Participants included seven students, seven academic supervisors and five workplace supervisors. The clinical context therefore focused on the perspectives of only three stakeholders. No consideration was given to the possible influence colleagues, managers, clinical supervisors or the specifics of the clinical work had on learning. In order to address the research questions listed earlier, consideration of all major stakeholders within the learning milieu and exploration of their influence on CS was required. Interestingly, Dewar and Walker (1999) conclude that there was a gap between the academic programmes and the experiential learning that took place in the clinical context.

Cowley (1995) provides an overview of the use of illuminative evaluation to investigate professional development and change in a learning environment going through a period of transition. Cowley was asked to enter the organisational life of an inner-city community healthcare provider to examine factors that were 'internal' to the organisation, seek information about how best to obtain and use nursing advice throughout this work setting and explore the more general learning that occurred in a community healthcare provider.

She recognised that, in addition to listening to what people said, it was important to explore what happened in practice. Data were collected through observation, focus groups involving locality managers, neighbourhood nurse managers and community nurse practitioners and by interviewing 'key informants' individually. However, some of the focus groups comprised both managers and practitioners, thereby threatening the freedom of participants to express their particular views. Cowley (1995) could have arranged separate focus groups specific to job title, for example managers and practitioners, and used other meetings to 'observe' the interactions between managers and their staff. In the context of the present study, it was felt necessary to create an atmosphere where stakeholders would feel at ease in discussing their particular view.

Cowley (1995) chose illuminative evaluation to investigate the learning that occurs in a healthcare organisation. She argues that the project uncovered evidence to suggest that hierarchical constraints, which had supposedly been dissolved, continued and remarks: 'such an organisation seems more likely to inhibit than promote development in professional nursing practice' (p. 973). Similarly, the present study sought to explore CS in the organisational context of teams in the Mental Health Directorate (MHD) of a Primary Care Trust. Consequently, the design and data-gathering methods had to be sufficiently comprehensive to explore the complexity of factors influencing the ways mental health nurses engage with CS.

A small proportion of the studies conducted in nursing using illuminative evaluation have included aspects of the case-study approach. Smith *et al.* (1995, p. 248) investigated four centres (case sites) and conclude that 'the combination of illuminative evaluation and case study benefit from yielding data high in validity'. Six case studies were used in Dewar and Walker's (1999) investigation of work-based learning within a post-registration community health nursing degree programme. According to Dewar and Walker (1999), case studies aided an in-depth exploration of the different perspectives of stakeholders.

Case-study research, like illuminative evaluation, was developed as an alternative to the experimental paradigm. It has been described as an empirical inquiry, investigating a phenomenon in its real-life context and using multiple sources of evidence (Yin, 1994). The data-gathering techniques for case-study research are similar to those used in an illuminative-evaluation investigation; data from interviews, observation and documentation create a case-study database. In the context of the present study, in order to illuminate how team climate, ways of working and clinical priorities influence the engagement in CS, it was felt that the analysis and reporting of results could be assisted using a series of case studies. This is clarified later.

Critical appraisal of using illuminative evaluation is scarce. There is a paucity of discussion in the nursing literature concerning the merits of illuminative evaluation. Crotty (1990, p. 375), after conducting an illuminative-evaluation study, concludes: 'the illuminative evaluation approach taken for this study has provided information in order to give a comprehensive understanding of the course in reality'. However, as with other nurse researchers (e.g. Chambers, 1988; Smith *et al.*, 1995; Hamlin, 1996; May *et al.*, 1997; Mhaolrunaigh and Clifford, 1998), there is an absence of critical debate on the benefits and shortcomings of illuminative evaluation. An investigation using the illuminative-evaluation approach for the investigation of learning outwith an educational institution should provide a critique of its appropriateness.

SUMMARY OF METHODOLOGICAL CONSIDERATIONS

Illuminative evaluation belongs to a group of approaches described as developmental evaluation (Øvretveit, 1998). It is acknowledged that it moves away from the experimental evaluation paradigm and is not concerned with cause and effect but rather with description and interpretation. Nonetheless, illuminative evaluation has an important contribution, particularly when what is being evaluated is unclear, may change throughout the duration of the study or where there is uncertainty about its effects and uncertainty about what causes or influences these effects. Its strengths arise from the illumination of an alternative perspective. Illuminative evaluation brings into focus other stakeholders' views, describes methods for gathering these and creates a comprehensive description of the evaluated in its natural context.

DISCUSSION OF DATA-COLLECTION TECHNIQUES

In this section, the methodological considerations and the decisions taken relating to data-gathering strategies for the current study are addressed. Chapter 5 describes the study design and provides further detail on how these methods are to be incorporated.

Parlett and Hamilton (1972) note three stages in an illuminative evaluation: observation, inquire further and seek to explain. They suggest that the three stages might overlap and 'functionally interrelate' (Parlett and Hamilton, 1972, p. 18). Within this three-stage structure, an information vignette can be constructed using data collected from four areas: interviews, observation, questionnaires and tests, and documentary and background sources (Parlett and Hamilton, 1972, p. 18). In order to answer the research questions posed earlier, I had to consider appropriate data-collection methods. Would a single method, for example in-depth interviews, capture all the required data or, as Parlett and Hamilton (1972) suggest, would a combination of interviews, observation, questionnaires and documentary evidence be necessary?

INTERVIEW

Parlett and Hamilton (1972) support the adoption of the research interview in order to investigate the impact of an innovation. They clarify this approach by stating that 'instructors and students are asked about their work, what they think of it, how it compares with previous experience; and also to comment on the use and value of the innovation' (Parlett and Hamilton, 1972, p. 20). Incorporation of the qualitative interview is ubiquitous in illuminative-evaluation research (e.g. Shapiro et al., 1983; Melton and Zimmer, 1987; Robinson, 1991; Cowley, 1995; Dewar and Walker, 1999). Nonetheless, when deciding if the qualitative interview should be incorporated, choices had to be made concerning which format would address the issues relevant to the study.

The focus group, which has been used in previous illuminative-evaluation projects, was considered. While the focus group does have certain advantages, for example it is inexpensive, flexible, elaborative and capable of producing rich data (Streubert and Carpenter, 1999), its use in other illuminative evaluations has highlighted some potential problems. A similar concern is raised from Nicklin's (1997b) research into CS in a general hospital environment. In this study, supervisors and supervisees participated in the same focus groups. The nature and complexity of the issues being explored precluded this sort of use of focus groups in the current study. It was felt that including several stake-holders in the same group would limit the sharing of individual perspectives. Furthermore, the number of participants would be insufficient for the consideration of separate focus groups for specific stakeholders. The suggested optimum number is between six and eight members (Basch, 1987; Kitzinger, 1995).

As an alternative, the individual in-depth interview was considered to be useful in answering the questions particular to this study. The qualitative interview is known for its ability to capture some of the richness and complexity of the subject matter under investigation (Rubin and Rubin, 1995). According to Brenner *et al.* (1985), the central value is that the interview dialogue offers the opportunity for immediate clarification, further elaboration and probing. It allows both the interviewer and respondent to explore the meaning of the questions and answers involved. As new perspectives emerge, the researcher can pursue those lines of inquiry, because the goal of the investigation is to understand the experienced phenomenon as fully as possible. However, it is the participants' perspective on the phenomenon that should unfold and not how the researcher views it. Knowledge is arrived at inductively, leading from specific observations to the identification of general patterns (Robson, 1993).

It has been suggested that there are some aspects of the qualitative interview that are a challenge, for example the ability to establish rapport and elicit information from participants. Nevertheless, according to Grbich (1999), the interviewer is of central importance to the interview process. The quality and substance of the data collected depend largely on the quality of the relationship between researcher and participant. It was felt that my non-hierarchical position within the Trust's MHD would be salient to the development of such a relationship and my role as a clinician would allow me to align closely to the research participants. My non-involvement in the provision of research participants' CS would also be relevant. The work of Berg *et al.* (1994), Nicklin (1997b) and Severinsson (1995), where researcher also functioned as supervisor, could be challenged for this reason. In these studies, researchers investigated the effectiveness of an intervention they themselves had provided. Ultimately, this may have created researcher and subject bias. The current study set out to unravel the complexities of the supervisory endeavour. Its objective in this regard could have been compromised by dual relationships.

The interpersonal effectiveness of the interviewer is also significant. Throughout the research interview, steady eye contact should be maintained and, as Barker (1996, p. 227) suggests, 'appropriate to what amounts to a deep conversation'. My experience working as a mental health nurse and as an accredited cognitive psychotherapist aided the development of an effective interpersonal style. I considered myself skilled in facilitating clinical interviews and was confident in my ability to transfer those interpersonal skills into a different interview context. These skills enabled me to engage participants in describing their supervisory experiences. Additionally, 14 years' experience as a clinical supervisor to a wide variety of healthcare professionals including mental health nurses, psychiatrists, clinical psychologists and psychotherapists helped me refine these interpersonal skills. It was important for me to extrapolate these further into a research domain.

Since the study's research questions focus on specific aspects of CS, it was necessary to incorporate some structure to the interview. Severinsson and Hallberg (1996) used an interview guide, which contains useful questions. Nonetheless, four of their questions may have led into discussions that had no relevance to the interviewee's own experience. It was felt that in view of the explorative nature of the current study it was necessary for the interview guide to contain open-ended questions. The interview guide was developed from relevant issues emerging from the literature review, and particularly some of the previous work that focused on 'good characteristics'. However, the study's research questions were the main source of guidance.

The semi-structured qualitative interview was considered to be capable of providing data necessary to address the probing and explorative questions stated earlier (p. 41). From these interviews, it would be possible to gain some understanding of participants' experiences with CS. Clarity concerning a range of issues would be achieved. Involving clinical supervisor and supervisees would facilitate a more comprehensive understanding of CS and a more balanced perspective. Previous supervision research has tended to focus on one group of practitioners (e.g. Pesut and Williams, 1990; Severinsson, 1995). This has resulted in the unfolding of a distinct, biased perspective. Consequently, in the present study, the views and opinions of other stakeholders were required. Since it was important to identify organisational factors, which may have been impacting on the delivery of CS, it was necessary to include practitioners who had a management function in the teams.

However, a further concern emerged that relates to the self-report nature of interview data. This was particularly relevant to the question: 'How do the interactions between clinical supervisor and supervisee influence the content of clinical supervision?' It is well known that research participants may have a personal understanding which could give rise to a biased understanding of issues. Using a protective front or disclosing a public rather than a private view affects the trustworthiness of the 'truth' that emerges (Grbich, 1999). Conducting separate individual interviews with various stakeholders may not eradicate the unfolding of particular biases. Furthermore, the current project was concerned with illuminating a deeper and more comprehensive understanding of what happens during CS sessions, what supervisees and clinical supervisors discuss and how they interact. It demanded methods that would complement the strengths of the semi-structured qualitative interview but counteract its limitations.

AUDIO-RECORDING OF CLINICAL SUPERVISION

In order to address question two – 'How do the interactions between clinical supervisor and supervisee during supervision sessions influence its content?' – it was felt necessary to turn attention towards the routine engagement of CS sessions. A greater focus on the interactions during supervision sessions and observing what clinical supervisors and their supervisees actually talk about was required. It is argued that a systematic observation of interactions during CS is essential to an investigation that proposes to uncover aspects of the supervisory process. This is an aspect of CS that has received minimal attention in the nursing community. However, this generated a dilemma concerning how such interactions would be observed.

When adopting an illuminative-evaluation approach, Parlett and Hamilton (1972) stress the value of observation as part of the data-gathering armoury. These observations could provide additional information that might not be uncovered from interviews. Parlett and Hamilton (1972, p. 19) state: 'the language conventions, slang, jargon, and metaphors that characterise conversation within each learning milieu, can reveal tacit assumptions, inter-personal relationships and status differentials'. Nonetheless, it was felt important not to invade clinical supervisors' and supervisees' private discussions in a direct, obtrusive and potentially negative fashion – other, less intrusive, observation strategies were required. It is noteworthy that participants in Malin's (2000) study refused the direct observation of their supervision sessions.

Using video-recording equipment would have provided an opportunity to observe verbal and non-verbal interactions. However, this was deemed too problematic. First, video-recording equipment is considered almost as intrusive as direct observation and therefore poses similar detrimental consequences. Second, I was doubtful of participants' willingness to have interactions video-recorded, particularly in relation to maintaining their anonymity. Third, the use of such equipment is complicated and therefore there is greater potential for losing data. Goin and Kline (1974), Shanfield et al. (1993), Keller et al. (1996) and Milne and Westerman (2001) video-recorded supervision sessions during their research on supervisory interactions. However, these researchers make no reference to its ability to capture non-verbal aspects of communication. On the contrary, results from their research concentrate solely on the significance of verbal communication. It appeared that studying the verbal exchanges between clinical supervisor and supervisee could be a valuable means of exploring aspects of this interpersonal relationship.

As an alternative, the use of audio-recording equipment to capture verbal interactions was considered to be a valid and reasonable compromise. It is acknowledged that observation of the verbal interactions is restrictive. Nonetheless, this technique could be helpful in answering the question: 'How do the interactions between clinical supervisor and supervisee influence the content of clinical supervision?' Moreover, it was felt that audio-recordings, because they are first-order data, would allow a close exploration of supervision as it happens (Grbich, 1999) and may be less inhibiting than video-recording.

Audio-recordings of therapy sessions for the purposes of CS have wide use in the psychotherapy, psychology and counselling professions (Liese and Beck, 1997; Bernard and Goodyear, 1998; Rosenbaum and Ronen, 1998; Temple and Bowers, 1998). In this context, audio-recordings enable the review of verbal aspects of therapist–client interactions. Equally, the paralinguistic aspects of these communications can be examined. Scaife (2001) points out that the use of audio-recordings of therapy sessions can be beneficial in supervision and suggests that this method may offer particular advantages over other methods. For example, audio-recordings provide an opportunity for a detailed review of client–therapist interactions and therefore a benefit for exploring supervisor–supervisee interactions in the current study.

Audio-recording nurse–patient interactions has been successful in previous nursing research. Macleod Clark (1982) and Wilkinson (1991) found that recording nurse–patient interactions provided relevant data on verbal exchanges. These researchers identified 'facilitating' and 'blocking' behaviours used by nurses during their interactions with patients. In a more recent study, Whyte and Watson (1998) describe the use of a radio microphone to record nurse–patient interactions. Audio-recordings have been used in previous supervision research. Severinsson (1995) analysed data derived from the transcriptions of audio-recordings of group supervision sessions in her 'good characteristics of supervision' investigation. Holloway (1982) and Holloway and Wampold (1983) used the audio-recordings of supervision to investigate supervisor–supervisee interactions. In this work, researchers have used only a proportion of the total number of audio-recordings available. In the present study, it was necessary to request that participants' audio-record sessions over a considerable period of time and explain that all sessions would be utilised for analysis.

It was felt that audio-recording supervision sessions would enable the gathering of data for an in-depth analysis of the full extent and context of verbal and paralinguistic aspects of the interactions between clinical supervisor and supervisee. From this, an exploration of the influence each participant's verbal behaviour had on the other would be possible. Further, the subjective accounts that participants shared during interviews concerning the content and potential changes could be considered in a more comprehensive way with the addition of indirect observation data.

However, it was acknowledged that audio-recording CS sessions would not be without difficulty. There is little mention in the literature of nurses using audio-recordings of nurse–patient interactions or supervisor–supervisee interactions for the purposes of their own supervision. This may relate to how CS has been interpreted in nursing. Since its introduction, concerns have been raised that CS is nothing more than a means of surveillance or monitoring

(Platt-Koch, 1986; Carthy, 1994; Burrow, 1995). According to Wilkin *et al.* (1997), one of the reasons for nurses resisting CS is the perception of it being a management-monitoring tool. In acknowledging nurses' unfamiliarity with the audio-recording technique, I recognised the necessity for the provision of a thorough explanation.

A further concern about recording sessions relates to how participants would feel about having their supervisory discussions audio-recorded. Supervisees take certain issues to supervision for discussion because they feel safe and secure with their clinical supervisor having access to such information. Normally, the dialogue between supervisor and supervisee is private and confidential. Similar to Malin's (2000) investigation, I was concerned that participants would be reluctant to hand over audio-recordings of their supervision for research purposes. Finally, it was possible that these audio-recordings may not allow an exploration of routine transactions. One possible disadvantage of using observation during research, according to Grbich (1999), is that participants may develop extra layers of covering, thus limiting access to the insider view. Participants, knowing that these sessions were being audio-recorded, could function in ways that were quite remote from how they normally engage in supervision.

One way of overcoming this phenomenon, known as the Hawthorne effect, was to explain that I was interested in participants' current supervisory practices and to emphasise the importance of uncovering things as they are. By engaging in the research process without preconceived notions of what to expect, the possibility of participants making assumptions about what was the 'right' thing to do was minimised. Thus, participants would have had difficulty in behaving in the 'right way', since they were unfamiliar with what this 'looked like'. The longitudinal nature of the study and the prolonged indirect observation helped to minimise this. Patton (1990) stresses that prolonged engagement reduces the likelihood of behaviour resulting from the 'observer effect'.

Another strategy used to minimise the 'observer effect' was to give participants ownership of a tape once a supervision session had been audio-recorded. Participants were encouraged to listen to the recording and then decide whether or not to submit the tape. Participants were assured safe storage of their tape recordings, that access to the recordings was limited to a secretary, transcribing some of the tapes, and myself and so their anonymity would be secured. Despite the possibility for untrustworthy information, this component of the data-gathering strategy was considered to be valuable.

It was understood that the combination of the qualitative interview and the audio-recording of CS sessions could contribute to achieving some of the study's objectives. However, self-report interview data are retrospective; data derived from the audio-recordings are subject to the researcher's interpretation. Consequently, it was felt that such data might not allow complete coverage of the objective: 'Identify the uses of individual clinical supervision by mental health nurses working in a Primary Care Trust'.

CLINICAL SUPERVISION SESSION RECORD

Previous research investigating the content of CS has generally relied on retrospective, self-report data (see Chapter 2). I wanted to provide supervisees the opportunity to document the content of their supervision sessions on an ongoing basis during the study.

The administrative aspects of CS, for example record-keeping, have received little attention in the literature. However, issues relating to this are now beginning to be addressed. Bond and Holland (1998), Power (1999) and Driscoll (2000a) favour the recording of some information relating to the content and structure of CS. When notes are made, they should, according to Bond and Holland (1998), include general subject headings, have the agreement of the supervisee and supervisor and not contain any information that might identify either the client or the colleague. Using such records as an aide-memoire is an obvious benefit. Additionally, keeping records of supervision is believed to help clarify what the supervisee wants to discuss; over time they can highlight recurring themes (Cutcliffe, 2000b) and uncover supervisee development (Power, 1999; Driscoll, 2000a).

It is therefore perhaps surprising that a written record of CS sessions has not been a common data-collection technique in previous supervision research. I thought it could be advantageous to collect such documentation if they were being kept or, if not, to incorporate a session document. By maintaining a supervision session record, supervisees could document their understanding of the issues discussed during a particular supervision session. Furthermore, analysis of such data could illuminate recurring themes and supervisee development.

However, I was aware that, if the development of a document were required, it would need to correspond with current thinking on record-keeping as detailed previously. Brevity was an important concern. The eventual document took into consideration these issues and assisted in a more comprehensive exploration of objective one, listed earlier. The session document provided participants the opportunity to outline the agenda for the session, give a description of what topics were discussed, detail any actions suggested following the discussion and document the date and time for the next session. Participants were discouraged from writing specific personal information on clients or colleagues, or any other information that could identify individuals.

OTHER DOCUMENTS RELATING TO CLINICAL SUPERVISION

In the original account of the illuminative-evaluation method, Parlett and Hamilton (1972) point out the necessity to consider the 'instructional system'. CS, in the present study, was an innovation that had educational underpinnings and which had been in use in a healthcare context that was investigated. Since the study did not focus on a purely educational innovation and its implementation into an academic setting, the 'catalogue' (Parlett and Hamilton, 1972), as described earlier, was modified. For the purposes of this study, organisational or team policy statements relating to CS, educational descriptors of CS courses that participants had attended and the wider CS literature pertaining to nursing were considered to be the 'instructional system'. It was felt that these documents would have to be analysed since their contribution to the ways in which CS was adopted in the research location could not be overlooked. By incorporating these related documents question three – 'How do the organisational factors affect the supervisory process?' – would be answered more comprehensively.

CRITICAL INCIDENT JOURNAL

While an illuminative-evaluation study emphasises data derived from interviews and observation, it does not refrain from conventional 'paper and pencil' techniques. Parlett and Hamilton (1972, p. 22) explain that 'Besides completing questionnaires, participants can also be asked to prepare written comments on the programme; to go through check-lists; or compile work diaries that record their activities over a specific period of time.'

Related to this were concerns of how consideration could be given to question four: 'What changes are reported from this experience of individual CS?' As previously highlighted in Chapter 2, the expectations relating to the impact CS has on nurses' work are considerable. Restricting participants to completing a specific questionnaire, which relates to any of the reported expectations, has been shown in previous research to be of limited value. I felt that it was necessary for supervisees to be given the opportunity to elaborate on aspects of their experience. A diary or journal, as suggested by Parlett and Hamilton (1972), seemed an appropriate strategy.

It was Flanagan (1954) who first devised the critical incident technique for gathering information concerning effective and ineffective behaviours in certain contexts. This method evolved during World War II for the purpose of studying what qualities were necessary to become a good combat pilot (Runeson et al., 2001). In the original paper, the critical incident technique is described as: 'A set of procedures for collecting direct observations of human behaviour in such a way as to facilitate their potential usefulness in solving practical problems' (Flanagan, 1954, p. 327).

Since its first description, the critical incident technique has been used by a number of researchers, in a variety of occupational groups, to investigate aspects of practice and to evaluate performance. It was Benner (1984) who popularised this method as a research strategy and suggested it would assist in delineating the link between the art and science of nursing. The critical incident technique is now used widely in nursing research (e.g. Cormack, 1983; Parker et al., 1995; Minghella and Benson, 1995; Austin et al., 2000; Kemppainen, 2000; McDonald and Glover, 2000; Mitchell, 2001). The range of issues being investigated highlights the flexibility of this method.

But what are critical incidents? Tripp (1993, p. 8) argues that critical incidents are produced by the way situations are perceived; they are interpretations of the significance of the event. Clamp (1980, p. 1755) suggests that critical incidents are: 'Snapshot views of daily work of the nurse and by examining them the effects of care on patients can be seen, and interactions between colleagues can be highlighted.'

Any experience that a practitioner encounters is potentially a critical incident and therefore a situation on which they can reflect. The actual incident can be an event that, to others, may seem to be nothing more than an ordinary experience (Wilkin, 1998). It is the individual's appraisal of the incident that makes it significant. Alternatively, it can be an incident where the experience did not go to plan or one that went well. An incident could be one that identifies the contribution of CS to mental health nurses' work experience. Norman et al. (1992) notes from research eliciting high- and low-quality nursing care from patients and their nurses that respondents were unable to give a detailed account of such incidents. Nonetheless, they argue that validity may be established by the fact that participants appeared to recount what actually happened as they saw it; what they said was clearly important to them. Thus, a major strength of the critical incident technique is that it usually results in a context-specific description of what nurses do, rather than a description of what participants think they do or what they think they should do. It gives a description of actual events and is therefore more concerned with the real, rather than the imagined.

Teasdale et al. (1998) and Malin (2000) use a variation of diary-keeping in their investigations of CS, gathering evidence on its impact using critical incident forms. In Teasdale et al.'s (1998) study, participants were asked to share information on one recent incident; both supervised and unsupervised nurses (n = 211) returned 156 forms and responses were mostly patient-focused. The critical incident journal provided participants with the opportunity to describe their out-of-session experiences and their relatedness to supervisory discussions. Requesting that participants maintain a critical incident journal over an extended period of time could have developed this approach. Furthermore, contrary to Teasdale et al.'s (1998) primary intention, data from the critical incident journal aided further exploration of supervisees' experience of supervision. Teasdale et al. (1998) highlight that negative feelings arose in 17% of the critical incident forms, for example participants expressed dissatisfaction with their supervisor.

Critical incident journals do have a disadvantage. Richardson (1994) stresses that the utility of the critical incident journal is dependent on participants' motivation. Similarly, the level of information participants wish to disclose will influence entries (Dachelet et al., 1981; Mitchell, 2001). Thus, when using a journal, crucial and relevant data may be overlooked because participants deem them unimportant or judge them irrelevant to the researcher's quest. To reduce the likelihood of this, the provision of a detailed explanation of the critical incident journal is recommended. Nonetheless, it was anticipated that a critical incident journal would provide another dimension to the supervisee's perceptions of how supervisory discussions impact on the supervisees' clinical practice, that is their work experiences beyond the CS session.

SUMMARY OF DATA-COLLECTION TECHNIQUES

The previous sections provide a discussion of the illuminative-evaluation approach and consideration of appropriate data-gathering techniques felt suitable to answer the research questions listed previously. A fuller description of how particular data-collection techniques were incorporated into the project is provided in Chapter 5. The merits and limitations of using the illuminative-evaluation approach are considered in Chapter 8. While Chapter 4 provides a full discussion on the analytic frameworks that were considered suitable for this project, data analysis in illuminative evaluation will now be discussed.

DATA ANALYSIS

In considering the questions central to the study, decisions were made to adopt certain data-gathering techniques into this illuminative-evaluation project. It was acknowledged that the data generated from the individual semi-structured in-depth qualitative interview, audio-recordings of supervision sessions, a CS session record, other supervisory documents and a critical incident journal would be copious and textual, qualitative data. An analytic approach capable of guiding the analysis of these data was required.

While they allude to the gathering of qualitative data, Parlett and Hamilton (1972) omit any suggestion or guidance on data analysis. In the absence of such advice, I felt it was important to consider how other nurse researchers who had conducted an illuminative-evaluation study had gone about analysing similar sorts of data.

CONTENT ANALYSIS

Although content analysis does occur in qualitative research, the enumerative approach is more widespread. According to Grbich (1999), this approach is characterised by the development of 'objective' accounts of the content of verbal, visual or written texts. After codes and categories are identified, the frequency of occurrence of particular units is measured. Issues of 'validity', 'reliability' and 'generalisability', as defined within the quantitative paradigm, are important issues. Chambers (1988), Hamlin (1996) and Mhaolrunaigh and Clifford (1998) describe the analysis of data in their illuminative-evaluation projects using this approach. Yet, this approach of analysis would appear incongruous with Parlett and Hamilton's (1972) justification in the generation of qualitative data. An illuminative-evaluation study, and the data-gathering techniques adopted, is used in order to gain a rich, context-specific understanding of an innovation. Parlett and Hamilton (1972) stress that:

> Research on innovation can be enlightening to the innovator and to the whole academic community by clarifying the processes of education and by helping the innovator and other interested parties to identify those procedures, those elements in the educational effort, which seem to have had desirable results. (p. 9)

Inherently, the emphasis is on description and interpretation rather than measurement and prediction. The research conducted by Dewar and Walker (1999) refers to the development of categories and the emergence of key themes, suggesting some form of thematic analysis.

It was important to adopt an approach for the analysis of the present study's data that was compatible with the underlying premise of illuminative evaluation. The present investigation set out to describe the content, structure and reported changes resulting from CS. In order to gain an appreciation and understanding of the complexity of processes intrinsic to the phenomenon, an approach that would facilitate the emergence of integral themes was required.

THEMATIC ANALYSIS

Philip Burnard (1991), one of nursing's most prolific writers, developed an approach for the analysis of textual data. The qualitative data analysis method 'thematic content analysis' is an adaptation of Glaser and Strauss's grounded theory approach and from various works on content analysis (Glaser and Strauss, 1967; Babbie, 1979; Fox, 1982; Berg, 1989). Burnard (1991) suggests that thematic content analysis aims to produce a detailed and systematic recording of the themes and issues together under a reasonably exhaustive category system. Since its first description in the nursing literature, the technique has been used extensively in nursing research (e.g. McGaughey and Harrison, 1994; Gijbels, 1995; Breeze and Repper, 1998; Rush and Ouellet, 1998; Knott and Latter, 1999; Sloan, 1999; Samuelsson et al., 2000; Whittaker and Ball, 2000; Wikberg et al., 2000). In this work, the approach has been used to analyse semi-structured and unstructured interview data. It was felt that thematic content analysis could be useful for the analysis of data generated from the other data-gathering techniques integral to the current study.

However, rather than refer to this analytic method as 'thematic content analysis' (Burnard, 1991), I use the term 'thematic analysis' since it depicts more accurately how it has been used in this study. It is also notable from Burnard's (1991) original description that 'content analysis' in its traditional sense is not an aspect of 'thematic content analysis'. The goal in the present investigation was to obtain a comprehensive and exhaustive cluster of categories. There was no need to quantify these categories, as would happen during a 'content analysis' (Grbich, 1999).

ANALYSIS OF VERBAL TRANSACTIONS

The exploration of the interpersonal interactions between clinical supervisor and supervisee was central to this investigation. In Chapter 2, some discussion was offered concerning the analytic frameworks used in previous research. The advantages and disadvantages of using one of these approaches, Blumberg's Interactional Analysis (BIA) framework (Blumberg, 1970), were considered. If this were adopted, comparison with similar research would have been possible. However, it was considered unsuitable for the present study. Instead, a framework capable of capturing nurses' verbal interactions during CS was necessary. Discussion and justification for the use of such an analytic framework is provided in Chapter 4.

THE LEARNING MILIEU

Question three – 'How do the organisational factors for clinical supervision affect the supervisory process?' – was concerned with uncovering some of the contextual factors influencing the provision of CS. As illustrated later in Chapter 5, the MHD in the Primary Care Trust was subdivided into six service sectors. Each sector was divided into specific clinical areas. Each of these areas functioned as an independent unit and was identified as a 'team'. Each team had its own specific geographical area, client group, clinical priorities, working practices and membership. Thus, the clinical context (team) where mental health nurses worked was understood as the 'learning milieu'. In order to gain a comprehensive and accurate understanding of participants' experiences of CS, data were organised and analysed in accordance with 'team' boundaries. Consequently, in order to illuminate how team climate, ways of working and clinical priorities influenced the engagement in CS, it was felt that the analysis and reporting of results could be assisted using a series of case studies with each team being regarded as a case. It was imperative to develop an accurate description and interpretation of how each team incorporated CS.

CONCLUSION

This chapter began with a statement of the general aim, research questions and objectives of the investigation. Following on from this, a case for an illuminative evaluation investigating individual CS in mental health nursing was presented. The challenges in adopting this evaluative approach and the methodological considerations relating to the present study have been discussed. The following chapter provides justification for the incorporation of an additional analytic framework.

4 Analytic Framework

INTRODUCTION

During the development of the initial proposal for the study, it was apparent that in order to address the overall aim and research questions posed in Chapter 3 theories relating to interpersonal interactions required consideration. The question 'How do the interactions between clinical supervisor and supervisee during supervisory sessions influence the content of clinical supervision?' (p. 41) is central to developing an understanding of the processes of CS. In Chapter 2, the Blumberg Interactional Analysis (BIA) framework (Blumberg, 1970), an analytic framework that had been used in previous supervision research, was critically appraised and deemed unsuitable for this study. Two further theories were considered: Peplau's theory on Interpersonal Relations in Nursing (Peplau, 1952) and Heron's Six Category Intervention Analysis (Heron, 1976). In this chapter, a rationale for electing to use Heron's analytic framework in preference to Peplau's theory will be presented.

PEPLAU'S THEORY OF INTERPERSONAL RELATIONS

In 1952, Hildegard Peplau, a nurse theorist and psychoanalyst from North America, published her book *Interpersonal Relations in Nursing*, in which she described the phases of the interpersonal process, roles in nursing situations and methods for studying nursing as an interpersonal process in the context of the nurse–patient relationship. According to Peplau, nursing is a therapeutic activity that can be viewed as an interpersonal process because it involves two or more people with a common goal. I was curious to explore whether her theory of interpersonal relations would be applicable to the context of the interpersonal processes integral to the supervisory relationship.

Peplau identifies four sequential phases that occur during nurse–patient relations: orientation, identification, exploitation and termination (Peplau, 1952). In the initial phase, the nurse and patient meet as total strangers; they orientate themselves to each other and develop a rapport. Towards the end of the orientation phase, the nurse and patient begin to clarify problems. During the identification phase, the patient responds selectively to those professionals who can meet his or her needs. Problems are identified and the patient decides who can assist in resolving these concerns. Following on from this, in the exploitation phase the patient makes use of all available services. In the resolution phase, the patient and nurse have worked together to meet the patient's needs and so the relationship can be terminated. As the nurse helps the patient work towards a resolution to their problems, these phases may overlap and interrelate (Peplau, 1952).

Peplau believes that the nurse–patient relationship is purposeful and goal-centred. The nurse's function is to help to reduce any anxiety experienced by the patient by channelling energy towards interpersonal growth. The nurse, adopting a number of roles, and the patient progress through the various phases to achieve this growth (Peplau, 1952). The roles are determined by the nature and stage of the patient's problems and include the roles of stranger, teacher, leader, counsellor, resource person and surrogate. When in a teaching role, the nurse may impart knowledge in reference to the patient's needs. In a counselling role, he or she may help to resolve problems that are interfering with the patient's ability to live effectively (Belcher and Fish, 1985). Peplau argues that the nurse should approach the patient as a complete person and be concerned with the 'total growth' of the patient's personality.

According to Peplau, in the interpersonal-relations paradigm, the nurse–patient relationship has a communicative character. Peplau differentiates between 'social talking' and 'therapeutic conversation' and suggests that nurses should not talk to the patient in the same way that they would speak to family or friends. The nurse's speech must lead to therapeutic effects and promote the patient's long-term well-being (Peplau, 1989). Accordingly, Peplau's theory of interpersonal relations is generally argued as useful for the creation of a therapeutic nurse–patient relationship where the patient, experiencing an illness, is assisted in the forward movement towards creative, constructive and productive community and personal living. Perhaps not surprisingly, Peplau's interpersonal theory has proved beneficial in clarifying nurses' contribution during therapeutic nurse–patient relationships (Martin, 1987; Lemmer, 1988; Gauthier, 2000).

Nonetheless, this important strength limits the model's use in the current study. Peplau argues that her framework has benefits for nurses when they engage in a therapeutic relationship with patients. The four phases depicted by Peplau relate to the purposeful creation of a therapeutic relationship between nurse and patient. The roles of stranger, teacher, counsellor, leader, surrogate and resource person in this context may be relevant and appropriate. However, in the context of CS where the interpersonal relations involve a colleague-to-colleague context, some of these roles were unsuitable. The potential for CS to provide a therapeutic purpose for supervisees, for example, remains a debatable issue in nursing. While there are a few scholars who appear to support CS having an intentional therapeutic purpose (Chambers and Long, 1995; Jones, 1995b; Hadfield, 2000), others are dismissive of this (Yegdich, 1998, 1999a; Power, 1999; Cotton, 2001).

A further limitation concerns the phases of Peplau's developmental framework. The phases (orientation, identification, exploitation and termination) are a significant aspect of the model. For the purposes of this study, some of these phases were not applicable, particularly the orientation and termination phases. Question two of the present study sought to identify interpersonal transactions between clinical supervisor and supervisee in a relationship that already existed. Thus, relationships were established; the orientation phase would most likely have already been worked through. Equally, since it was expected that supervisory relationships would continue long after this investigation was complete, the termination phase was also considered to be inappropriate in the current study.

Peplau's model of interpersonal relations has been criticised because it places too much emphasis on process at the expense of structure (Walsh, 1991). Peplau's model does not offer a structured assessment format when working through the orientation and identification phases. This creates the potential for patient problems to be overlooked or formulated incorrectly. Furthermore, the theory gives no explanation or detail concerning possible nursing behaviours for the exploitation phase. It was felt that this would cause difficulty when analysing supervisor behaviours in the context of these phases.

Peplau's theory is grounded in a generous assumption in that the value, and particularly the therapeutic gain for the patient, when nurses adopt the interpersonal-relations model is dependent on nurses engaging therapeutically with patients. Her theory was borne from working as an advanced nurse therapist having trained as a psychoanalyst in North America in 1953 under the supervision of Frieda Fromm-Reichman (Barker, 1999). Thus, interpersonal-relations theory developed from observations in the psychiatric clinics of North America of advanced nursing practice supplemented with training in psychoanalytic psychotherapy. Can this theory and its assumptions transfer to mental health nursing in the UK? Research investigating the therapeutic work of mental health nurses without additional psychotherapy training provides substantial evidence to suggest that they cannot (Altschul, 1972; Cormack, 1976; Bray, 1999). Moreover, Peplau's model fails to provide guidance on how to identify nurse–patient interactions that are not therapeutic. In the present study, I made no assumptions concerning whether supervisory interactions would be helpful or otherwise. I wanted to explore and describe the nature of such interactions. The analytic framework adopted in the present study would need to be comprehensive enough to allow for the delineation of both helpful and unhelpful behaviours.

At a superficial level, Peplau's theory of interpersonal relations might be considered relevant as an analytic framework for this study. However, because its focus is on particular developmental stages of interpersonal relations and is primarily concerned with the purposeful engagement in a therapeutic relationship and the adoption of specific roles, it was felt to be unsuitable for the current study.

My familiarity with Peplau's theory developed when I commenced a Diploma in Professional Studies in Nursing in around 1989. As part of a module, 'Systematic Nursing Care', I studied, amongst other nurse theorists' work, Peplau's interpersonal-relations framework. A further module facilitated my introduction and understanding of Heron's analytic framework. In 1989, I began working in a psychotherapy unit, where interpersonal relationships and related skills were important aspects of the work. Studying Heron's work introduced me to Philip Burnard and Peter Morrison's investigation of nurses' interpersonal skills. Following a short introduction to the clinical application of Six Category Intervention Analysis, I began to integrate it into my own therapeutic work.

A description and explanation of Heron's analytic framework will follow. Thereafter, a discussion on its use in previous nursing research investigating the interpersonal skills of nurses and its incorporation as a CS model will be presented. From this, I will justify its use as an analytic framework in the current study.

SIX CATEGORY INTERVENTION ANALYSIS

Heron's Six Category Intervention Analysis is a conceptual model that was initially developed to progress the understanding of interpersonal relations, and specifically to assist the delivery of interventions within a helping paradigm. Since 1975, the model has been influential in guiding mental health nurses in their interactions with patients (Hammond, 1983; Chambers, 1990; Ashmore, 1999). Burnard (1985, 2002) popularised Heron's work for general nursing settings in his book *Learning Human Skills*. He suggests that the nurse who develops competence in the six categories of intervention could become an effective helper in a broad range of interpersonal contexts. In addition to clarifying its clinical application, Burnard has used the model as a conceptual framework investigating nurses' perceptions of their interpersonal skills (Burnard and Morrison, 1988, 1991; Morrison and Burnard, 1989). More recently, it has been put forward as a suitable model to guide the delivery of CS in nursing (Chambers and Long, 1995; Cutcliffe and Epling, 1997).

According to Heron (1976), the interpersonal relationship takes place between a practitioner and client. A practitioner is defined as anyone who offers a professional service to a client; so the term refers equally to a doctor, psychiatrist, psychotherapist, nurse, lawyer and teacher, for example. The client is the person who chooses to involve him- or herself in the service that the practitioner is offering in order to meet a need the client has identified.

Heron (1989) extends this primary account of practitioner and client roles. In the first extension, the terms 'practitioner' and 'client' can be applied in formal, occupational settings, where two people in any organisation relate to each other in terms of their work roles and where one person intervenes with another. Hierarchically, in line-management terms, they can be on either the same or different levels. Interventions in this context may be about work, discipline, career advice or even about personal matters that have some impact on work (Heron, 1989). In the second extension, the terms 'practitioner' and 'client' can be applied to non-formal and non-professional settings, whenever one person is assuming an enabling role for another, for example from one friend to another, lover to lover or colleague to colleague. In each of these interactions, one person is the listener or facilitator and the other is the talker, the one dealing with some specific issue.

Heron's framework progresses (see Table 4.1) from Blake and Mouton's (1976) diagnosis and development matrix, which comprises five categories: acceptant, catalytic, confrontation, prescription, and theories and principles. The focus of intervention between Blake and Mouton (1976) and Heron (1989) differs. When describing the work of Blake and Mouton (1976), Heron (1989, p. 7) explains: 'Their focus is primarily on interventions in organisational life as organisational development consultants. Mine is primarily on one-to-one interventions from practitioner to client.'

Blake and Mouton's (1976) matrix is intended for the analysis of interventions made in management consultancy, whereas Heron's framework is concerned with, primarily, one-to-one interventions between a practitioner and a client during a variety of helping exchanges.

Table 4.1 illustrates the categories and how they are divided into authoritative and facilitative interventions. Authoritative interventions are those that enable the practitioner to maintain some degree of control in the relationship, giving guidance and instruction to the client, whereas facilitative interventions allow the locus of control to remain with the client. Authoritative interventions are neither more nor less useful and valuable than the facilitative ones (Heron, 1989). Their appropriateness is dependent on the nature of the practitioner's role, the particular needs of the client and the content or focus of the intervention; it is the specific context that makes one intervention more or less beneficial than another.

According to Heron (1989), an intervention is a piece of verbal and/or non-verbal behaviour that is an aspect of the practitioner's service to the client.

Table 4.1 Six Category Intervention Analysis

Authoritative categories	Facilitative categories
prescriptive	cathartic
informative	catalytic
confronting	supportive

Throughout the framework manual, an emphasis is placed on the practitioner's verbal behaviour including the paralinguistic elements of speech. Heron argues that verbal behaviour can be described in three different ways.

- **verbatim:** the form of words used as an intervention, for example the practitioner says to the client, 'I think you should read some chapters from Melanie Fennel's book';
- **linguistic:** a description of the form of words used, for example the practitioner suggests some reading material;
- **intention:** the intervention is understood in terms of what the practitioner wants to achieve, for example to suggest a useful reading source.

The six category system describes six basic kinds of intention a practitioner can have when working with a client. Prescriptive interventions seek to influence and direct the behaviour of the client and include offering advice and making suggestions. To be informative is to offer information or instruction. Heron (1989, p. 38) states that 'informative interventions seek to impart to the client new knowledge, information and meaning that is relevant to their needs and interests'. Confronting interventions directly challenge the rigid and maladaptive ways that limit the client. A confronting intervention tells an uncomfortable truth, 'but does so with love, in order that the client concerned may see it and fully acknowledge it' (Heron, 1989, p. 45). Cathartic interventions assist the client to abreact painful emotion, for example grief, fear and anger. The interventions are pitched at a level of distress that the person is ready to deal with. Interestingly, Heron claims that cathartic and confronting interventions were those on which participants at his workshops rated themselves weakest. Catalytic interventions include encouraging further self-exploration, self-directed living, learning and problem-solving in the client. Lastly, to be supportive is to validate or confirm the worth of the client's person, qualities, attitudes or actions.

While Heron claims that the six categories are exhaustive of the major sorts of intervention any practitioner needs to offer in relation to clients, he points out that the list of interventions for each category is not exhaustive. Instead, in his publications he offers a comprehensive catalogue of interventions for each category (Heron, 1989, 1990, 2001).

In addition to describing helpful interventions, the framework also highlights strategies that can be considered degenerate and perverted (Heron, 1989). He elaborates:

> To say that an intervention is degenerate, in the sense intended here, is not to say that it is deliberately malicious or perverted (I deal with this type later); but rather that it is misguided, rooted in lack of awareness – lack of experience, of insight, of personal growth, or simply of training. (Heron, 1989, p. 149)

Four degenerate interventions are described: unsolicited, manipulative, compulsive and unskilled. An unsolicited intervention occurs when, without being asked, the practitioner starts to interact in a particular way with the client without any agreement, negotiation or permission, for example advising that the client do something when this has not been asked for or offering therapy when this is not appropriate to the task in hand. Manipulative interventions are motivated by the practitioner's self-interest regardless of the interests of the client; the practitioner gets what they want out of the interaction. Heron argues that compulsive interventions can be punitive, colluding or evasive and are rooted in the practitioner's unresolved psychological material. Lastly, unskilled interventions result from the practitioner's incompetence in interpersonal skills.

While degenerate interventions are rooted in a lack of awareness, lack of experience, lack of personal growth or a lack of training, perverted interventions are, according to Heron (1989), something darker. Perverted interventions are malicious, intentionally harmful and, in their execution, the practitioner sets out to do damage to the client. Heron suggests that such interventions are, in usual circumstances, nothing to do with normal practitioner–client interactions.

This interpersonal-relations framework did not develop from empirical research (Heron, 1976). Inspired by the work of Blake and Mouton (1976), Heron developed Six Category Intervention Analysis between 1973 and 1974 while he was running courses for experienced general practitioners, training them to become trainers of young hospital doctors entering general practice (Heron, 2001). He recounts:

> We evolved a set of behavioural categories that was relevant, when appropriately applied, both to the role of trainer and to the role of doctor. It then became clear it had universal application, and it has since provided the basis for interpersonal skills training in a wide diversity of social roles. (Heron, 2001, p. 1)

While working as a psychotherapist, group facilitator and trainer, Heron has revised and extended the model (Heron, 2001). Since its inception, there have been few studies that have attempted to validate its theoretical propositions. Instead, Heron (1990) argues that the overall legitimacy of his framework is a matter of ongoing experiential research. To date, few published studies have used the six category analysis to underpin research in the area of interpersonal relations. Yet it appears to hold some value in being incorporated in these types of investigation, particularly in the context of mental health nursing. When describing his category system, Heron (1989, p. 15) emphasises the fact that: 'The six categories per se and the sorts of interventions that fall under them do not entail any particular theoretical perspective coming from any school of psychology or psychotherapy.'

This has relevance for mental health nursing, since the possibility of dissonance between the practitioner's therapeutic orientation, for example solution-focused-brief therapy and the categories in Heron's framework, is minimised (Chambers, 1990). The six category framework, according to Heron, could be used as an analytic tool to compare and contrast the therapeutic practice of different psychotherapeutic methods.

Several nurse theorists have put forward a formulation that considers the therapeutic relationship as a central focus for nursing (Peplau, 1952; Orlando, 1961; Travelbee, 1971). O'Brien (2001) clarifies how the importance of a therapeutic interpersonal relationship between nurse and client in mental health nursing has developed during the last century. However, as suggested previously, research findings relating to mental health nursing in the UK seem to challenge this assertion. But while the therapeutic integrity of mental health nursing has been repeatedly questioned (Towell, 1975; Cormack, 1976; Martin, 1992; Gijbels, 1995; Robinson, 1996; Sullivan, 1998; Sainsbury Centre for Mental Health, 1998; Bray, 1999), this body of evidence tells us little about what does or does not happen during actual interpersonal relations between mental health nurses and the clients for whom they care. Heron's framework might be a useful method to investigate the delivery of interpersonal transactions used by mental health nurses regardless of the practitioner's particular therapeutic persuasions. Furthermore, it could also illuminate what is not happening during such interactions in mental health nursing.

NURSES' INTERPERSONAL SKILLS

In previous studies that investigated nurses' perceptions of their interpersonal skills, participants were asked to rank the six category items in response to how skilled they perceived themselves to be generally (Burnard and Morrison, 1988) or when working with patients (Morrison and Burnard, 1989; Ashmore and Banks, 1997).

Burnard and Morrison (1991) tested the reliability of their earlier work by using a different method of collecting data. Participants were asked to complete a rating scale, rating the six category items to correspond with how skilled they perceived themselves to be while talking to patients in a professional nursing setting. From a matrix consisting of rows and columns in which each row represented a respondent and each column represented a category of analysis, Burnard and Morrison (1991) were able to calculate mean rating scores for each of the categories. From this, Burnard and Morrison (1991) were able to rank the six categories in terms of the dimension 'least skilled – most skilled'.

The rank order supportive, informative, prescriptive, catalytic, cathartic and confronting is generated in Burnard and Morrison's (1988, 1991) and Morrison and Burnard's (1989) investigations. That is, these nurses perceived themselves as more skilled in using supportive (facilitative) and informative (authoritative) and prescriptive (authoritative) interventions. Conversely, research participants felt less skilled in being able to elicit patients' self-discovery (catalytic), facilitate the expression of strong and painful emotion (cathartic) and confront unhelpful patient behaviour (confronting). Burnard and Morrison (1989) acknowledge, as possible limitations of these studies, the difficulty in identifying participants' therapeutic intentions after the event, subject bias and the use of a forced-choice ranking exercise. Findings from this work support Heron's observation that participants on his workshops generally rate themselves weakest on cathartic and confronting interventions.

Heron's (2001) theory for this concerns the lack of emotional competence and resulting repression of painful emotions, for example grief, fear and anger. He explains:

> We do not learn techniques of controlling the distress emotions of grief, fear and anger non-repressively, nor the techniques of releasing them through aware and intentional catharsis, or of transmuting them by spiritual practices. In short, we do not as yet have any education and training of the emotions. (Heron, 2001, p. 75)

Nurses confront additional barriers to the effective care of patients' emotional distress; professional and organisational practices denigrate these issues (Dartington, 1993). Nurses are frequently faced with people in distress, and such work is not straightforward. But the nature of how nursing work is organised – its workload, the nature of patient problems, the throughput of patients, the competing demands on nurses' time – does not allow sufficient space to acknowledge and care effectively for patients' emotional needs. The delivery of cathartic interventions demands a level of interpersonal competence and sufficient time to facilitate catharses of emotion. This provides a possible explanation for nurses rating themselves weakest on cathartic interventions. Furthermore, perhaps nurses in these studies had a negative perception of confronting interventions and consequently rated themselves unfavourably in this category.

Morrison et al. (1991) subjected the findings of their survey of 117 trained nurses (Burnard and Morrison, 1991) to further statistical analysis. When using Smallest Space Analysis, Morrison et al. (1991) reveal unexpected patterns in the way the six category intervention items may be interrelated. The researchers suggest that the interventions could be considered in terms of two groups, those that involve the expression of emotion: cathartic, catalytic and confronting, and those that are more dispassionate: prescriptive and informative interventions. The supportive category is related to all other categories; supportive interventions underpin the other two groups. Morrison et al. (1991) find no empirical support for Heron's authoritative/facilitative division. In acknowledging the representation of CS in the nursing literature as a supportive resource for the supervisee to combat the stresses associated with nursing work and to develop knowledge and skills with the goal of improving patient care, examples from all six categories might be uncovered from an analysis of clinical supervisor–supervisee interactions. However, the organisational context may have some influence on how participants of CS interact.

A more recent study (Ashmore and Banks, 1997) used the same research instrument developed by Burnard and Morrison (1988, 1991) and Morrison and Burnard (1989) in an attempt to test the reliability of Burnard and Morrison's earlier findings with student nurses. They also hoped to make comparisons between their own study of qualified staff and Burnard and Morrison's (1991) study. A convenience sample of 311 student nurses undertaking a Project 2000 diploma course was introduced to Heron's framework. Each student was then asked to rate themselves on each of the six categories to correspond with how skilled they perceived themselves to be when interacting with patients. The rating scale procedure devised by Burnard and Morrison (1991) was followed. The student nurses perceived themselves as most skilled in the use of supportive, prescriptive and cathartic interventions and least skilled in informative, catalytic and confronting interventions. Thus, students from a Project 2000 course perceived themselves to be more skilled in facilitative interventions than authoritative ones, a change from previous findings. Nurses also continued to rate themselves weakest in confronting interventions.

It is notable that in all the previously mentioned studies what has been identified has been nurses' self-perceptions of how skilled they are in the use of interventions from Heron's framework. The results may have been influenced by the participants' relationship with the researchers (subject bias). That is, were nurses' responses to the rating scale influenced by the researchers and so they rated themselves high on supportive, prescriptive and cathartic interventions because that seemed to be the 'right' thing to do? Alternatively, a limited understanding of the interventions in each category may have influenced their responses. The researchers state: 'Respondents were introduced to Heron's six category intervention analysis, a brief description being given of each of the categories followed by a period of familiarization and clarification' (Ashmore and Banks, 1997, p. 338).

A brief explanation of this detailed and comprehensive, but complex, framework could result in various misunderstandings. Ashmore and Banks (1997) do question the accuracy of these self-perceptions in relation to actual everyday clinical nursing skills competence. Data obtained from practitioners' everyday clinical practice would have been a valuable addition to this study and would have enhanced the validity of the results. It would appear that Heron's framework remains to be incorporated in an investigation exploring the ways in which nurses engage with their patients during their day-to-day practices.

The significance of findings from previous studies has been limited as a result of using only participants' self-perceptions. As highlighted by Heron (1989), the framework has the potential as an analytic tool to explore practitioners' interpersonal behaviours in specific work-related contexts. So far, nursing, including the mental health speciality, has overlooked the value of

Heron's model in this regard. In addition to analysing the day-to-day work of mental health nurses, using the framework in this manner would also provide an opportunity to challenge its theoretical assertions. For example, can a helping exchange be confined to only one of the six categories, and can all helping exchanges be subsumed into six domains? Furthermore, gaining some appreciation of the types of supportive, prescriptive, cathartic, informative, catalytic and confronting interventions conveyed by nurses would be useful. Exploration of the impact of particular intervention categories requires empirical investigation. Although Heron (1989) provides descriptions of helping interventions, their impact and influence on interpersonal relations should be investigated in the context of CS.

HERON'S FRAMEWORK AND CLINICAL SUPERVISION

Heron's framework has been adopted as a supervision model in the nursing literature (e.g. Johns and Butcher, 1993; Chambers and Long, 1995; Fowler, 1996c; Cutcliffe and Epling, 1997; Driscoll, 2000a). As stated earlier, the framework has been used extensively in various professions as a structure for guiding interventions during helping relationships (Chambers, 1990). However, Heron illustrates how this template is applicable to the supervisory endeavour:

> In the first extension, the terms 'practitioner' and 'client' can be applied in formal, occupational settings, where two people in the same organisation are relating in terms of their work roles, and where one person is intervening in relation to the other. (Heron, 1989, p. 8)

Cutcliffe and Epling (1997) emphasise the enabling and therapeutic process that develops through the use of confronting interventions and claim that such interventions are not at odds with the supportive nature of CS. Rather than being regarded as a hostile attack, Cutcliffe and Epling (1997) suggest that confronting interventions should be viewed as offering a gift – a gift with the capability of increasing understanding and insight for the supervisee. These authors state that the therapeutic value of confronting interventions in the context of psychotherapy can be transferred to the supervisory experience and argue that the same therapeutic benefits that arise as a result of therapy can arise in a CS session.

On the other hand, Chambers and Long (1995) advocate an emphasis on the facilitative category and, in particular, supportive interventions. While Chambers and Long agree with Heron that none of the intervention categories is better than any other, they place more significance on the facilitative styles. In their description of a 'facilitative model of supportive clinical supervision' Chambers and Long (1995, p. 312) give encouragement to the adoption of supportive, cathartic and catalytic ways of intervening but make no reference to Heron's remaining categories. This particular approach to CS has received constructive comment on two counts. First, it demonstrates a conceptual error whereby CS is confused with providing therapy. Second, as a supportive approach, the strategies are misguided (Yegdich, 1999a).

It would appear that these writers advocate the use of only certain aspects of Heron's framework. Adopting Heron's framework in this way perhaps undermines its basic premise. Heron (1989, p. 14) proposes that 'there is no real hierarchy among the categories. No one of them is in principle good or bad in relation to any other. In the abstract they are of equal value.' The nature of the practitioner's role, the particular needs of the client and the focus of the helping relationship determine their importance. If we return to the funda-mental purpose of CS depicted in the psychotherapy literature, the develop-ment of therapeutic competence (Doehrmann, 1976; Loganbill *et al.*, 1982; Watkins, 1990; Bernard and Goodyear, 1998; Kilminster and Jolly, 2000), and recall the interpersonal focus detailed in definitions found in the nursing lit-erature (Chapter 2), the potential contribution of all six categories is obvious. In the case of CS where the clinical supervisor attempts to progress the super-visee's therapeutic proficiency, disregard for either the authoritative or facili-tative interventions may, in fact, undermine the dynamism of this framework. Similarly, the expectations resulting from participation in CS as depicted in the nursing literature (Chapter 2) highlight the potential value of all six cate-gories. In learning new ways of working with patients, supervisees' therapeu-tic competence could be progressed by a clinical supervisor using any of the six categories of intervention. In support of this approach, Fowler (1996c) offers all categories of the framework as a structure for clinical supervisors. He gives an example for each of the intervention categories, suggesting the framework offers the clinical supervisor six ways of taking CS forward.

Heron's (1989) framework as a model for CS has been subjected to research in the UK. Devitt (1998) explores the nature of the supervisory relationship and the labour of supervision through the eyes of the supervisor, using a grounded theory approach. Four supervisors working in acute paediatrics, intensive care and anaesthetic directorates participated in the study. Analysis of the data from a focus group, self-reported reflective diaries and in-depth interviews generated five sub-themes, which together have been conceptu-alised as a three-stage trajectory of the clinical supervisory relationship. Despite having an initial agreement that the use of Heron's framework would be limited to four of the six categories, confronting, cathartic, catalytic and supportive (mainly facilitative interventions), prescriptive and informative interventions (authoritative interventions) were used most frequently. Specific examples of these interventions are not given.

These data confirm previous results from the work of Burnard and Morrison (1988) and Morrison and Burnard (1989) that suggest nurses favour authoritative ways of interacting with patients. It is interesting that the par-ticipants in Devitt's (1998) study highlighted a preference for authoritative interventions when working with colleagues. No information was available concerning what grade of staff these participants (junior ward sisters) were supervising. No similar analysis of the ways mental health nurses use the categories in CS has been undertaken, and it is inappropriate to assume a similar preference is adopted in this branch of nursing.

HERON'S FRAMEWORK AS AN ANALYTIC TOOL

Heron (1989) proposes that his framework would be a useful means of analysing interactions between practitioners and their clients. This contribution has been supported, at least in principle, in nursing. Hammond (1983) shows how the framework could be used to either interpret nurse–client interactions or assist the nurse during a counselling session. More recently, Ashmore (1999) reinforces Heron's assertions and argues its value in comparing and contrasting different therapeutic practices. Following a comprehensive search of relevant databases, I was unable to identify any research that had incorporated Heron's framework for this purpose.

In considering the question 'How do the interactions between clinical supervisor and supervisee during supervision sessions influence the content of clinical supervision?', it was felt important to explore the nature of the interpersonal interactions. Heron's analytic method was considered a suitable framework for this endeavour. Following a review of the literature relating to how this framework has been adopted in previous interpersonal research, its value in this regard was confirmed. Having been incorporated to investigate nurses' self-reports on their interpersonal skills, it was felt appropriate to use the framework to analyse supervisor–supervisee interactions.

CONCLUSION

There are ongoing challenges regarding the therapeutic value of mental health nursing – a growing body of evidence suggests that the observed work of mental health nurses generally lacks any particular therapeutic intention (Cormack, 1976; Sainsbury Centre for Mental Health, 1998; Bray, 1999). However, none of this research illuminates what mental health nurses do, or do not do, when interacting with patients. Similar deficits exist in the CS literature; interpersonal interactions, which are potent in influencing changes in supervisee practice, remain enigmatic. In this chapter, the utility of Heron's framework to investigate the interpersonal interactions of mental health nurses as they engage in CS has been discussed. The current investigation, having this as its focus, would incorporate an analysis of actual nursing practice in the real world of healthcare. This would be in contrast to how the framework has been used in previous research. Furthermore, it would provide an opportunity to challenge the framework's theoretical standpoint.

5 Study Design and Methods

INTRODUCTION

In Chapter 3, the methodological considerations in adopting an illuminative-evaluation approach for this study were discussed. Parlett and Hamilton (1972) argue the case for the qualitative interview, observation, documentation and questionnaires as the standard methods in an illuminative-evaluation study. Previous nurse researchers have generally followed their guidance. As highlighted in Chapter 3, the methods chosen for the current project included a semi-structured qualitative interview, indirect observation using audio-recordings of CS sessions, CS documentation and a critical incident journal. This chapter will describe the overall design of the study, including a description of the learning milieux and instructional system, and how the research methods were used.

LOCATION

The study was conducted in the MHD of a large and widely dispersed Primary Care Trust in the west of Scotland. The MHD consisted of services for adult mental health, elderly mental illness (EMI), children and young people, learning disabilities and addictions. The adult services were further divided into area-wide services, including continuing care, resettlement, rehabilitation, an intensive psychiatric care unit, a day-resource centre and a day-activities team; North area services included three community mental health teams, a mental health day-resource centre and two hospital-based admission units; and South area services comprised three community mental health teams and two hospital-based admission units.

The EMI services were divided by geographical area and included hospital-based services, three day-care facilities and five community teams. At the commencement of the study, CS was underdeveloped in the majority of services within elderly mental health. Two community teams were providing opportunities for supervision.

Initially, two teams within adult mental health services (Case Site One and Two) and two teams from elderly mental health services (Case Site Three and Four) were the focus (see Figure 5.1). However, as a result of significant staff changes in Case Site Four, this team was withdrawn from the study. As previously highlighted, a clinical nurse manager (CNM) introduced CS to the

MHD of the Trust in 1985. Community mental health nurses, working in nursing teams, have had the opportunity of CS during the past 20 years. CS has continued to be utilised by those mental health nurses working in the community within multi-disciplinary mental health teams. The utilisation of CS within community-based resources created an ideal context for an investigation of CS in mental health nursing. Hospital-based mental health nurses, unlike their community counterparts, did not have the opportunity of CS and were therefore excluded from the study.

The community mental health teams (CMHTs) were set up with the intention to deliver comprehensive locally accessible mental health services for residents in the area they covered. They aimed to provide a multi-disciplinary approach to needs assessment and care management. Since their initiation in 1995, they have been offering a range of services that reflects the diversity of need in the local community. The main remit of these teams was to provide assessment, treatment, continuing care and support in the community to people with serious and enduring mental health problems with early intervention aimed at promoting and maintaining the mental health of individuals and their families and carers. People with less serious problems have also been offered this service. These multi-disciplinary teams included community mental health nurses, psychiatrists, social workers, clinical psychologists, occupational therapists and clerical support. Nursing staff provided the main human resources.

POPULATION AND SAMPLING ISSUES

The original description of illuminative evaluation gives little guidance on sampling (Parlett and Hamilton, 1972). The target population in the present study were those individuals who had a key influence in the provision of CS and those who incorporated it into their work practices. In order to address the questions central to this research, the population included senior management (senior manager (SM)), patient services managers (PSMs), middle management (team leaders (TLs)), clinical supervisors and supervisees working in, or responsible for, one of four teams.

This allowed a comprehensive exploration of the issues concerned with the study (Chinn, 1986; Munhall and Oiler, 1986). Purposive sampling as outlined by Robson (1993) is based on the researcher's judgement as to the typicality or interest of the case. Individuals are chosen because of their specific experience with the topic of interest (Streubert and Carpenter, 1999). My concern focused on developing a rich and context-specific description of the ways in which mental health nurses engaged with individual CS, and particularly the interactions between clinical supervisor and supervisee during supervisory sessions.

Using a purposive-sampling strategy, individuals from four teams from the MHD who fulfilled particular criteria (see below) and had experience with CS were invited to participate in the study. Supervisees were a particular focus of the present study and had to be working as a mental health nurse E-grade staff nurse (SN) at entry to study, working within one of the four teams from the two service areas and receiving CS at entry to the project. This specific level of practitioner was chosen for two main reasons. First, previous supervision research in nursing has tended not to focus on a particular grade of nurse. This makes it difficult to contemplate the relevance of such findings to specific grades of practitioners. Second, since emphasis has been placed on the provision of CS for D- and E-grade practitioners (Teasdale *et al.*, 1998), an exploration of the experiences of practioners working at this level was relevant. At the commencement of the study, clinical supervisors worked within one of the four teams; while not a prerequisite for their inclusion, all were G-grade charge nurses (CNs). The TLs managed the day-to-day running of the teams. The PSMs were responsible for a particular section of the MHD, for example adult mental health services in the North sector. The SM was identified as being central to the introduction of CS in 1985, and it was decided to request her participation in the study to gain an appreciation of her perspective on CS.

CASE SITES, PARTICIPANTS AND THEIR ROLE IN THE TEAM

Figure 5.1 illustrates the teams as cases, the participants involved in the study at its commencement and their function in the team. Participants' names have been changed to preserve their anonymity.

CASE SITE ONE

Case Site One was a community-based day hospital serving a rural area in the west of Scotland. During this investigation, the remit of the day hospital changed; its priority moved from providing treatment for a broad range of mental health difficulties towards working with patients suffering from severe mental illness. In a policy statement, the service was described as being an integral and essential component of the overall mental health service spanning hospital and community care for adults from 16 to 65 years of age. The aims of the service included:

- to provide treatment for those with significant mental illness in a day-hospital setting;
- to provide an alternative to acute hospital admission;

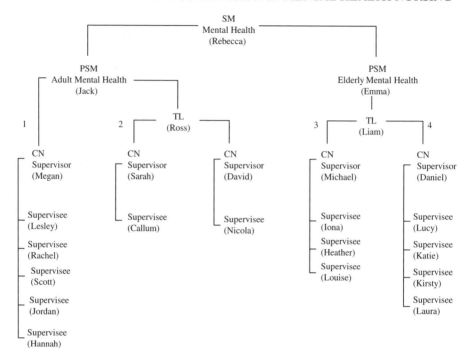

Figure 5.1 Case Sites, participants and their function at the study's commencement.

- to link with acute inpatient services and facilitate early discharge from hospital;
- to work jointly with CMHTs and support them in their management of complex cases.

Following this transition, a flexible programme of care delivered in groups was regarded as a key factor in its provision of services. In accordance with the Framework for Mental Health Services in Scotland (Scottish Office and DoH, 1997) individuals suffering from serious mental illness, at varying stages of their illness trajectory, were prioritised. Additionally, a satellite service had the task of delivering group programmes of care for people not necessarily suffering from serious mental illness in various community-based health facilities. While team members initiated this service development, CMHT colleagues contributed to the programmes of care. Patients received care in their own community rather than having to attend the team base, which might have required considerable travelling.

Nursing care was organised using a named-nurse system. SNs could have a caseload in excess of 40 patients, for whom they would be expected to conduct an initial assessment to identify needs, present their findings to the team and suggest a daily programme of varied activities. Skills-based groups, for example assertive skills, anxiety management and life skills, were the main format for the delivery of care. Nurses would arrange to meet with their patients to review this care package on a regular basis. Occasionally, in addition to a programme of varied activities, nurses would provide individual-therapy sessions.

A proportion of the team members had reservations concerning the changes that were being implemented to service delivery. Consequently, there was a great deal of effort expended by management and medical staff in order to maintain hierarchy in this team. The junior nursing staff (E grades) were subjected to the power and controlling aspects of the hierarchy. The influence that this exerted on the provision of CS is illuminated later in Chapter 7.

Staff Complement for Case Site One

CN (G grade)	Megan
SN (E grade)	Lesley, Rachel, Scott, Jordan, Hannah, Holly, Gillian and Georgie (plus two not participating)
Occupational therapist	(3)
Psychiatrist	(2)
Social worker	(1)
Dietician	(1)
Physiotherapist	(1)
Reflexologist	(1)
Pharmacist	(1)
Administrative staff	(2)

Participants and their team role

At the commencement of the study, all qualified nursing staff and relevant managers agreed to participate in the study. This included Rebecca (SM), Jack (PSM), Megan (CN – supervisor), Lesley, Rachel, Scott, Jordan and Hannah (SNs – supervisees). Case Site One did not have a TL; Jack compensated by visiting the team on a regular basis. As a consequence of service developments within the MHD, three supervisees (Rachel, Scott and Jordan) changed jobs and left the team during the study. After leaving the team, supervision was no longer sought from or offered by Megan for these SNs. However, the team recruited five new team members, of whom three agreed to participate in the research (Holly, Gillian and Georgie – Figure 5.2). Thus, only two of the ten SNs working in this team at the time of the investigation did not participate.

Rebecca, Jack and Megan each had a considerable length of experience working in mental health (>20 years); Gillian and Georgie had each worked

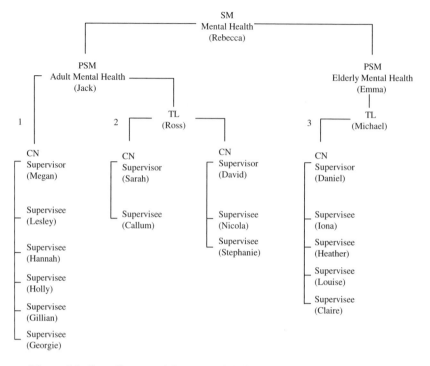

Figure 5.2 Case Sites, participants and their function at the study's completion.

in mental health nursing for approximately ten years; Lesley, Rachel, Holly, Scott and Jordan between five and ten years, and Hannah had less than five years' experience. In relation to continuing professional development, Georgie had been given the opportunity to undertake training in psychosocial interventions for people with psychosis. Rachel had undergone training in counselling at diploma level. Megan and Scott had taken an introduction to group therapy course. None of the other nurses had received any formalised training specific to the care programmes provided within the team base. Nonetheless, a small proportion of nurses (Lesley, Gillian and Hannah) had taken a module in group therapy at a local university.

CASE SITE TWO

Case Site Two was an adult CMHT situated in a large rural area in the west of Scotland. The main remit of the team was to provide assessment, treatment, continuing care and support in the community to people with serious and enduring mental health problems with early intervention aimed at promoting and maintaining the mental health of individuals from 16 to 65 years of age and their families and carers. People with less serious problems were also offered this service.

Nursing care was organised using a named-nurse system. SNs had a case-load of approximately 40 patients with a case mix of 60% enduring needs and 40% less-severe presentations. SNs would be expected to conduct an initial assessment to identify need, present their findings to the team and, following discussions, a programme of care would be established. If the team decided, the SN would have seen the patient for individual sessions. The delivery of nursing care during these individual sessions would include ongoing monitoring of mental health, the delivery of assertive skills or anxiety management and ensuring medication compliance. Some of the nurses provided group-based interventions, for example assertive skills, a lunch club or bereavement groups. Nurses would arrange to meet with their patients to review this care package on a regular basis. There was encouragement within the team for nursing staff to limit the extent of their contact with patients, particularly those having less serious mental health presentations.

The local population served by the team was divided into geographical areas, which were covered by a CN and SN. Each pair covered several GP practices and usually accepted patients for care referred from that particular area. This also served as a channel for good communication between the team and primary care staff.

Staff complement for Case Site Two

TL (H grade)	Ross
CN (G grade)	David and Sarah
SN (E grade)	Nicola, Callum and Stephanie
Nursing assistants	(1)
Occupational therapist (senior grade)	(1)
Clinical psychologist	4 sessions
Behavioural psychotherapist	2 sessions
Psychiatrist	9 sessions
Administrative staff	(2)

Participants and their team role

All of the qualified nursing staff in this team and relevant managers agreed to participate in the study. This included Rebecca (SM), Jack (PSM), Ross (TL), David and Sarah (CNs – clinical supervisors) and Nicola, Callum and Stephanie (SNs – supervisees). However, during the study, as a consequence of promotion, one of the supervisees (Nicola) left the team to take up post as charge nurse in a neighbouring adult CMHT. Nonetheless, David and this supervisee decided to continue with their supervisory arrangement. Despite Nicola being promoted to CN and moving to another team, I felt it was important to continue with data collection from this supervision pair. David continued to work within Case Site Two. This provided an opportunity to explore a supervisory experience that was unique in comparison to the routine supervision already available. Nicola was replaced in the team with Stephanie, who began to engage in CS with David. She agreed to participate in the study (Figures 5.1 and 5.2).

At the commencement of the investigation, Rebecca, Jack, Ross and Nicola each had considerable experience (>20 years) working in mental health; Callum, Sarah and David had worked in mental health nursing for between ten and 15 years, and Stephanie had less than five years' experience. In relation to continuing professional development, Ross, Nicola and Sarah had completed a diploma in community psychiatric nursing. David had completed a diploma in nursing and a degree in health studies. None of the nurses had received any additional formalised training specific to the care programmes provided within the team.

During the study, the team experienced a turbulent time. In addition to Nicola's departure, nursing assistants began working in the team and other team members encountered painful events in their personal lives. Ross, the TL, was given the additional responsibility of setting up a new service, thus reducing the time available for his own team. Consequently, there were high levels of distress and sickness absence, which ultimately impacted on the day-to-day workload of staff.

While hierarchy appeared to have some influence over the provision of CS in Case Site Two, management agendas were less prominent. Team members attempted to modify some of the controlling aspects of management that impacted on CS. Consequently, challenges to some of the rituals central to supervision became evident. Furthermore, team members appeared to battle against management agendas at a more general level. There was a strong effort to ignore the obvious differences in relation to professional membership and grading amongst team members.

CASE SITE THREE

Case Site Three was a CMHT, which was part of EMI services. The EMI services were divided into geographical area and included hospital-based services, three day-care facilities and five community teams. At the commencement of the study, CS was underdeveloped in the majority of services within elderly mental health. Two community teams were providing opportunities for CS. However, as explained later, following significant staff changes, Case Site Four (CMHT – EMI services) was withdrawn from the study. Case Site Three was based in a health centre in a rural area in the west of Scotland. The team adopted an open referral system for individuals over 65 years of age. Nursing care was organised using a named-nurse system. SNs could have a caseload of approximately 35 clients. There was considerable variation amongst nurses' caseload mix of clients with organic and functional presentations. The services this team provided included:

- an assessment of mental health needs;
- qualified nurses with specialist skills;
- individualised programmes of care;
- support;
- information and advice to clients and their carers;
- therapeutic treatments for specific mental health problems;
- group therapies;
- counselling;
- early intervention to promote and maintain the health of individuals;
- advocacy.

Staff complement for Case Site Three

TL (H grade)	Liam
CN (G grade)	Michael and Daniel
SN (E grade)	Iona, Heather, Louise and Claire
Nursing assistant	(2)
Occupational therapist	(1)
Psychiatrist	8 sessions
Administrative staff	(1)

Participants and their team role

All of the team's qualified nursing staff and relevant managers agreed to participate, which included the SM (Rebecca), the PSM (Emma), TL (Liam), CN (Michael) and three SNs (Iona, Heather and Louise). However, there were quite a number of staff changes during the initial stages of the study. Michael (clinical supervisor) was promoted to TL for that particular team; Liam had been the TL for both teams when the study commenced. Daniel (CN and clinical supervisor from Case Site Four) transferred to Case Site Three and started to provide supervision. At the same time, Claire was transferred into the team and began to receive CS from Daniel. She agreed to participate in the study (Figures 5.1 and 5.2).

At the commencement of the study, Emma, Liam, Michael and Claire each had considerable experience (>20 years) working in mental health nursing; Daniel, Heather, Iona and Louise each had approximately ten to 15 years' experience. In relation to continuing professional development, Michael had completed a diploma in community psychiatric nursing. Daniel had completed a degree in community psychiatric nursing and a diploma in bereavement counselling. Claire had completed a local course on psychosocial interventions for people with psychosis.

This team endorsed hierarchical functioning and lines of accountability. This appeared to have an impact on its provision of CS.

CASE SITE FOUR

Participants from this team included the PSM, TL, clinical supervisor (CN) and three SNs (supervisees). Daniel was transferred to Case Site Three as CN and clinical supervisor. Two SNs left the team. Following Daniel's move to his new team, no supervision opportunities were arranged for the remaining SNs. It was felt appropriate to withdraw this team from the study.

INSTRUCTIONAL SYSTEM

Earlier in Chapter 3, two concepts central to illuminative evaluation were described: the instructional system and the learning milieu. In traditional approaches to the evaluation of educational programmes, Parlett and Hamilton (1972) suggest there is a failure to recognise the 'catalogue' for what it is. The catalogue, or instructional system, is an idealised specification of a new programme and often contains grand objectives, a new syllabus and details of teaching techniques and equipment. While the concept of the 'instructional system' has most relevance in educational contexts, its usefulness can be justified in an investigation of the practice of CS. In this chapter, aspects of the instructional system relevant to this study are clarified.

In this study, the instructional system included a Trust document: 'Discussion Paper on Clinical Supervision for Nursing within the Community Health Care Trust' (Appendix One), a module descriptor for a CS module taught at a local university, and the recurring themes identified in the wider CS literature pertaining to nursing.

TRUST DISCUSSION PAPER

Appendix One presents the Trust discussion paper on CS and highlights the aspects of CS. However, to summarise, following an explanation of CS and presentation of audit results, key areas include a description of Proctor's supervision model and a suggestion that this would be a suitable framework for CS in the Trust and that CS is described as providing an opportunity for learning and the subsequent development of practice. The discussion paper reinforces that supervisees should have some degree of choice in selecting their clinical supervisor and that the clinical supervisor be separate from line-management structures.

While the working group recognised that some of the skills required of a clinical supervisor were skills considered to be requisite for nurses, further training to enhance these skills and learn how to apply them in the context of CS was clarified. Practitioners were made aware of the working group's vision of creating opportunities for formal preparation for the role of clinical supervisor.

The paper emphasises that each nurse within the Trust should be afforded, as a minimum, one hour of formalised CS every four weeks. It was expected that informal (ad hoc) supervision, which has always been practised by nurses, would continue; it would supplement formalised CS.

The usefulness of a supervision contract, which would outline roles and responsibilities of each participant, is described. Reviewing the contract at regular intervals (six-monthly) encouraged feedback on the usefulness of supervision and tensions in the relationship. Renegotiating this contract was thought to provide participants with the opportunity to decide if they wanted to continue or discontinue this arrangement. It was acknowledged that any discontinuation of the supervisory relationship was quite legitimate when either participant was dissatisfied with the experience and reparation was not possible.

In summary, the core strands of the discussion paper emphasise that CS should be distinct from line management and that CS, unlike managerial supervision, should be practitioner-driven. Accordingly, it is suggested that practitioners should have some degree of choice over their clinical supervisor. It is anticipated that clinical supervisors will not be allocated to practitioners. The development of professional skills through a process of reflective practice is identified as the main purpose of CS. The benefits of having a supervision contract with regular reviews of the usefulness of CS are also to be highlighted. In the likelihood of unsatisfactory CS, where reparation is not possible, it is suggested that alternative arrangements can be sought.

MODULE DESCRIPTOR

'Supervision for the Health Professions' is a level-three, 20-credit-point module and comprises 12 hours of lectures and 12 hours of seminars. These presentations include defining CS, models for supervision, its representation in nursing, discussions based on the conceptual and theoretical constructs of supervision, reflective practice, instruments for evaluating supervision and an overview of the empirical literature. In total, students have 24 hours of face-to-face, three-hours-per-week contact.

During the module, students are exposed to experiential learning by being encouraged to engage in three formats of CS: group supervision facilitated by the module leader, individual peer supervision with a colleague from their workplace and individual supervision with their line manager. Students have the opportunity to reflect on their experiences of supervision each week. Towards the end of the 12-week module, students are required to complete a written assignment, a reflective paper describing their supervisory experiences during the module.

The aim of this module is not necessarily to prepare practitioners for, the role of clinical supervisor; rather, students are introduced to, and prepared for, the experience of CS. Emerging ideas and findings from the conceptual and empirical literature are contemplated. It is hoped that course participants' awareness of the complexities concerning CS develop. Their experiences of implementing and developing their practice of CS are explored in a group. The module was included as an aspect of the instructional system since its broad aims and methods of teaching were considered as a further influence on how CS was practised by those participants who had undertaken the module. Several participants had completed this module.

RECURRING THEMES IN THE NURSING LITERATURE

The third aspect of the instructional system concerned the recurring themes emanating from the nursing literature. While the scope of influence of this component was regarded as less central as the Trust discussion paper or the module descriptor to the practice of CS in the research site, its contribution could not be overlooked.

Clinical supervision as a supportive resource

In Chapter 2, a plethora of alleged benefits relating to CS was presented. On reviewing the literature, it would appear that more emphasis is placed on some of these benefits than others. Certainly, CS as a supportive resource is widely acknowledged (e.g. Kaberry, 1992; DoH, 1993; Chambers and Long, 1995; Farrington, 1995; Cutcliffe and Epling, 1997; Wilkin, 1999; Claveirole and Mathers, 2003; Walsh et al., 2003). But Faugier and Butterworth (1994) expand the supportive function when they imply support refers to 'psychological support'. This transformation has been supported by a large-scale supervision project (Butterworth et al., 1997) and by Coleman and Rafferty (1995), Fowler (1996c), RCN (1999), Wilkin (1999), Rafferty (2000), Kopp (2001) and Veeramah (2002) when they propose CS as a means to reducing the level of stress, resolving personal issues and enhancing the emotional well-being of nurses. While the supportive ethos of CS is undisputed, the blurring of its supportive function and being therapeutic has been challenged.

Managerial agendas encroaching on clinical supervision

A frequently cited reason for some of the strong resistance towards CS in the UK concerns a fear of managerial agendas driving its practice (van Ooijen, 1994; Lyle, 1998a; Duncan-Grant, 2000a; Holyoake, 2000). In particular, there is concern that CS is nothing more than a management-monitoring tool (Wilkin et al., 1997). Gilbert (2001, p. 204) goes so far as to suggest CS is a 'method of surveillance disciplining the activity of professionals'. While some writers suggest that this contributes to the ineffective engagement in CS (Bowles and Young, 1998; Duarri and Kendrick, 1999; Power, 1999), others support a marriage of CS and managerial agendas (Fisher, 1996; Fursland, 1998; Docherty, 2000; Darley, 2001; Gray, 2001). Despite these tensions, it would appear that CS as practised in the UK is either a substitute for, or an extension of, managerial supervision (Gilmore, 1999).

In much of the empirical work carried out in general nursing settings, CS has been described as being management-led and provided by the supervisee's line manager (Swain, 1995; Butterworth *et al.*, 1997; Davidson, 1998; Teasdale *et al.*, 2001). A similar scenario is evident in research that has focused on mental health nursing (e.g. Scanlon and Weir, 1997; Sloan, 1999; Duncan-Grant, 2000b; Veeramah, 2002). In their fourth census of community mental health nursing in Northern Ireland, Brooker and White (1997) conclude that the most common relationship between clinical supervisor and supervisee is a managerial one. Findings from a recent survey (Kelly *et al.*, 2001) suggest that CS in Northern Ireland continues to be provided by a line manager. Senior managers and team leaders in Duncan-Grant's (2000a) research, where the supervisor was almost exclusively a line manager, regarded staff surveillance as an explicit aspect of CS. However, Jones and Bennett (1998, p. 21) assert that this opinion is not confined to managers when they state there is 'a need for mental health professionals to receive CS that builds in systems to monitor their practice'.

The broad scope of clinical supervision

As presented in Chapter 2, a multitude of alleged benefits of CS illustrate that its scope in the UK extends beyond being educational and supportive. These multiple interpretations have been challenged, for example Yegdich and Cushing (1998) question the controlling and therapeutic practices of CS in the UK. Yet, others have sought to expand its scope. Managerial agendas are evident when CS has been described as nothing more than risk management (Tingle, 1995), performance review (Swain, 1995) and caseload management (Gilmore, 1999). A therapeutic allegiance is illustrated when McEvoy (1993) reports that personal worries or problems at work could be discussed, Oliver (1995) encourages discussion of personal issues and Butcher (1995) recommends the discussion of staff relations. Others, for example Johns and Graham (1994), Morcom and Hughes (1996), Marrow *et al.* (1997), Kitchen (1999) and Clifton (2002), connect reflection and reflective practice to CS.

DATA-COLLECTION METHODS

In Chapter 3, the methodological considerations relating to an illuminative-evaluation approach and data-gathering strategies for the current study were discussed. In this section, how these data-gathering methods were incorpo-

Table 5.1 Study objectives and related data-gathering methods

To identify the uses of individual clinical supervision by mental health nurses working in an NHS Primary Health Care Trust.	Individual in-depth interview Clinical supervision session document Critical incident journal Audio-recording of supervision sessions
To explore and describe SNs' experiences of individual clinical supervision.	Individual in-depth interview Critical incident journal Audio-recording of sessions
To describe how the organisational provision of clinical supervision affects the ways in which the supervisory process is used.	Individual in-depth interview Background documents relating to supervision
To explore how the interactions between supervisor and supervisee during clinical supervision influence its content.	Individual in-depth interview Audio-recording of sessions Critical incident journal
To illuminate outcomes from the supervisory experience.	Individual in-depth interview Audio-recording of sessions Critical incident journal

rated in the current study is described. Table 5.1 details the data-gathering strategies for each of the study's objectives.

INTERVIEW

A semi-structured interview was used in this study and a process described by Patton (1990) informed and guided my approach in exploring participants' experiences with CS. The interview questions were contained in an interview guide with a specific focus on the issues central to the project. Although the sequence of questioning could vary, the interview guide ensured that I collected similar types of data from all participants. However, because of the range of informants, the interview guides did vary slightly for each level of participant (Appendix Two). All of the interview guides were evaluated for their comprehensiveness and relevance to the focus of the research in a pilot study, which is described in the next chapter.

Information sought from the PSMs and TLs included their perspectives on the purpose of CS, the system of CS made available and how it developed, their understanding of what happens during CS, the benefits and how these are demonstrated. Clinical supervisors were asked about their understanding of the ways in which CS is used, the structure of the supervision they provided, what issues were discussed, how they interacted with their supervisees during supervision and the benefits gained from their delivery of CS. Supervisees were asked about their perspective of CS, what they talked about, what factors influenced this, what they noticed about their clinical supervisor during supervision sessions, examples of good and bad supervision and the benefits they experienced as a result of CS.

Participants were encouraged to determine a venue for the interview suitable to them. The majority chose an office at their own team base that was conducive to interviewing without interruption or distraction; others opted for my own office, which was a considerable distance from their usual place of work. Several participants worried that our conversations might be overheard by other team members and therefore preferred the interview to take place away from their team base. Prior to the interview, I prepared by reading through the interview schedule. Participants were offered a cup of tea or coffee and I helped them settle into the interview by expressing my appreciation of their participation and reminding them of the importance of hearing about their experiences. The recording equipment was checked before beginning the interview by asking participants an icebreaker question. For example, I may have asked them to tell me about an aspect of their work that had gone well, a recent holiday or a favourite pastime. Back-up equipment, including a recorder, microphone, batteries and tapes, was always available. Providing all the equipment was working properly, the interview would begin. Interviews generally lasted between 45 minutes and an hour and 30 minutes.

To help maintain focus on exploring participants' supervisory experiences, I separated my clinical and research work. I arranged between two and three research interviews on the days set aside for this aspect of the study. My clinical work was conducted on other days. This prevented me from having to switch between therapist and researcher roles.

At the end of the interview, many participants commented on the usefulness of having taken part and were positive about this experience. They felt it had given them an opportunity to reflect on their supervisory encounters. Moreover, they were able to discuss aspects of their supervision and its impact on them, which until this interview had not been available to them. Many participants were astonished at how long they could talk on the subject. This may have occurred partly in response to the researcher conveying facilitative aspects of interviewing (Gordon, 1975) and an interest in their experiences. I did emphasise the significance of participants' experience, its importance to the study and attempted to understand their perspective of CS. At the conclusion of the interview, I completed a contact summary sheet making brief notes on the interview, first impressions and relevance to research questions.

At the commencement of the study, participants were working in one of two teams from the adult mental health services or in the EMI services. The diagrammatic representations (Figure 5.1 and Figure 5.2) illustrate the total number of participants in the study (n = 25) and their role in their respective team. All participants engaged in the semi-structured individual in-depth interview. A minority of participants were, however, interviewed more than once. This was as a result of new staff members joining each of the teams. I

Table 5.2 Interviews for each Case Site

Case Site One	Case Site Two	Case Site Three
13	11	10

returned to clinical supervisors to explore their approach with these new supervisees. Table 5.2 illustrates the number of interviews in each Case Site.

AUDIO-RECORDING OF SUPERVISION SESSIONS

This aspect of data collection concerned supervision pairs; the clinical supervisor and supervisee were the focus. Consequently, it required the consent and cooperation of both participants and could not occur without the agreement of both parties. My initial strategy, in keeping with Parlett and Hamilton's (1972) progressive focusing, involved approaching the clinical supervisor and supervisee as a pair. Following their separate individual in-depth interviews, I sought their informed consent for audio-recording supervision sessions. However, with late arrivals to the study and having gained consent for audio-recording supervision sessions from the clinical supervisors, I sought supervisees' informed consent for all aspects of the data collection.

It was important to clarify with participants that, once a session had been audio-recorded, the recording was their property. Participants were encouraged to listen to the recording before deciding whether or not to submit their tapes. Furthermore, they were encouraged to use the on/off switch to stop and start the tape if they did not want certain aspects of the discussion to be recorded.

Supervision pairs were asked to audio-record their supervision sessions over a 12- to 18-month period and encouraged to submit tapes consecutively. Supervision pairs were aware of their autonomy and freedom for deciding which tapes they submitted. Table 5.3 below highlights the supervision pairs from each team who agreed to participate in this aspect of the data collection and the number of tapes they submitted. A minority of participants declined to allow sessions being recorded. In total, 49 tapes were submitted collectively from eight supervision pairs.

From Table 5.3 it is clear there was some variation in the quantity of tapes submitted between supervision pairs and teams. The reasons participants gave for this included supervision sessions being cancelled, recording equipment not working properly, lack of audio cassettes, staff sickness and staff leaving the team and therefore supervision ceasing (Megan and Scott, for example). Participants informed me that all audio-recordings from their supervision sessions were submitted; no tapes were withheld from the researcher. A small number of tapes had sections of the recording deleted. Either participants

Table 5.3 Audio-recordings of supervision sessions

Case Site One		Case Site Two		Case Site Three	
Supervision pair	Number of tapes	Supervision pair	Number of tapes	Supervision pair	Number of tapes
Megan and Lesley	6	David and Nicola	10	Daniel and Claire	5
Megan and Scott	1	David and Stephanie	6		
Megan and Holly	7				
Megan and Gillian	10				
Megan and Georgie	4				
Totals	28		16		5

bringing their tapes to the researcher's office or the researcher collecting these from their respective team bases ensured the safe receipt of audio-recordings.

Audio-recording equipment

I sought guidance and advice from other qualitative researchers and audio-recording-equipment specialists concerning suitable recording devices. On their recommendation, Sony TCM-453V cassette recorders, Sony ECM-F8 microphones and TDK-120 (2-hour) tapes were purchased and used to audio-record the in-depth interviews and supervision sessions during the initial pilot study (see Chapter 6) and main study. The TDK-120 tapes were chosen for their ability to record material for an hour without interruption. Supervision pairs were given an explanation and demonstration of the recording equipment, and no major problems were encountered throughout the study.

CLINICAL SUPERVISION SESSION RECORDS

All supervisees were requested to keep a record of the issues taken to, and discussions during, their CS using a supervision session document (Appendix Three). Participants from Case Site Three had already been keeping a session document. Table 5.4 highlights the number of session documents submitted from each participant from each of the teams.

CRITICAL INCIDENT JOURNAL

All supervisees participating in the study were asked to keep a critical incident journal. It was intended to provide participants with the opportunity to

Table 5.4 Clinical supervision session records

Case Site One		Case Site Two		Case Site Three	
Lesley	9	Nicola	3	Claire	3
Rachel	1			Heather	2
Scott	3			Iona	4
Holly	10			Claire	9
Gillian	10				
Georgie	5				
Totals	38		3		18

illuminate how supervisory discussions impacted on their clinical practice, that is their work experiences beyond the CS session.

Rather than use the strategy as a stand-alone method for individual interviews, I incorporated a critical incident journal with other data-gathering approaches. Supervisees were sent instructions concerning their critical incident journal. This explanation was reinforced during face-to-face meetings. At the outset, participants were sent 12 sheets of carbon-copy paper and asked to send one copy to the researcher and keep the other (their journal). As part of my explanation, I stressed that the event or incident did not have to be dramatic but rather provoke deep thought and relate to their experience of CS. Participants were asked to remove any identifying information relating to their clients or colleagues not involved in the study. During a supervision session, supervisees are given the scope to reflect on aspects of their clinical work (Driscoll, 2000a). The critical incident technique provided participants the opportunity to reflect on their experiences of supervision. Supervisees were asked to keep a critical incident journal for the duration of the study.

One obvious disadvantage in using a critical incident journal is the time required for its completion. To minimise participants feeling burdened, I made no demands on the quantity of entries. Rather, I left decisions regarding the frequency of entries to participants' own discretion. Participants were reminded every three months throughout the duration of the study to submit their critical incident journal entries. A small number of critical incident journal entries was received.

I endeavoured to provide participants with adequate scope when completing their journal. I wanted to minimise the possibility of their contributions being influenced by their perceptions of my expectations. To reduce the likelihood of this, an explanation of their journal was provided. However, rather than give specific instruction on the information sought, the guidance was more general. I refrained from requesting examples of how CS had impacted on participants' work with patients, for example. Instead, I sought a description of any incident that had made an impact on them; it was the significance of the incident to them that I wanted to be the stimulant for their entries.

Table 5.5 Critical incident journal entries

Case Site One		Case Site Two		Case Site Three	
Lesley	5	Nicola	3	Claire	3
Gillian	1				
Holly	1				
Totals	7		3		3

Table 5.6 Data source and type from each Case Site

	Case Site One	Case Site Two	Case Site Three
Interviews	13	11	10
Audio-recordings	28	16	5
Session documents	38	3	18
Critical incident journal	7	3	3

SUMMARY OF DATA-COLLECTION METHODS

From Table 5.6, it is clear that Case Site Three has the smallest data set, particularly of audio-recordings. This is perhaps not surprising since only one pair agreed to have sessions audio-recorded. Data from this site is less comprehensive than Case Site One and Case Site Two. Therefore, a cautious interpretation of data from Case Site Three was necessary.

TRIANGULATION

The incorporation of different data-gathering techniques during an illuminative-evaluation study is thought to aid the uncovering of a more comprehensive perspective on the problem being investigated. Parlett and Hamilton state that:

> Equally no method is used exclusively or in isolation; different techniques are combined to throw a light on a common problem. Besides viewing the problem from a number of angles, this 'triangulation' approach also facilitates the cross-checking of otherwise tentative findings. (Parlett and Hamilton, 1972, p. 16)

Navigators use the term 'triangulation' to describe a technique of plotting a position using three separate reference points. Campbell and Fiske (1959) were the first to apply the navigational term to a research context. The metaphor is a good one because a phenomenon under study in a qualitative research project is much like a ship at sea. The exact description of the phenomenon is unclear. To gain progress and a clearer understanding about a particular phenomenon, researchers study it from a specific vantage point. From this, they learn additional information about the phenomenon. However, the information at this juncture is not precise. Researchers have to move to a different point to investigate the phenomenon further. The ultimate goal in choosing different perspectives is to help create a more comprehensive understanding of the phenomenon under investigation.

Combined with the semi-structured in-depth interviews from a diversity of participants, the CS session records, critical incident journals and the audio-recordings of supervision sessions constitute what Denzin (1989) describes as triangulation. In the present study, data triangulation (source, space and time) was used, whereby managers, clinical supervisors and supervisees were asked about their experiences of CS. The learning milieu in three Case Sites was compared and contrasted. Lastly, the audio-recordings of supervision sessions were conducted over a 12- to 18-month period. Methodological triangulation (across method) including interviews, session documents, critical incident journals and audio-recordings of supervision sessions was adopted in order to develop the comprehensiveness and completeness of the data. Similarly, analytic triangulation (Kimchi et al., 1991), which involves the use of two or more approaches to the analysis of the same data set, was incorporated. Comparing results of data analysed using differing qualitative analysing techniques to assess any similarity of findings enables researchers to note similar patterns and therefore verify findings. This collective can be thought of as an example of multiple triangulation (Denzin, 1989). He asserts: 'Multiple triangulation exists when a combination of multiple observers, theoretical perspectives, sources of data and methodologies are used' (Denzin, 1989, p. 310).

Multiple triangulation describes a combination of more than one type of triangulation within the same research design. Initially, researchers wrote of triangulation as though it were merely the use of multiple methods for the sole purpose of attaining confirmation (Denzin, 1970). However, this view has been extended to incorporate the purpose of 'completeness'. Jick (1979, p. 603) argues that triangulation can be something other than convergent validation. It can also capture a more complete, holistic and contextual portrayal of the unit(s) under study. The use of multiple sources is thought to uncover some unique variance that otherwise may have been neglected by a single perspective. It provides breadth and depth to an investigation. Jick (1979, p. 604) writes: 'In this sense, triangulation may be used not only to examine the same phenomenon from multiple perspectives but also to enrich our understanding by allowing for new or deeper dimensions to emerge.' This position has received support from Mitchell (1986), Corner (1991), Redfern and Norman (1994), Begley (1996) and Streubert and Carpenter (1999).

The metaphor of a group of visually impaired people describing an elephant based on the area they touch provides a good description of completeness. The most accurate description of the elephant comes from a combination of all the group members' descriptions. None of the individual descriptions would be complete or accurate. Combining data from the vantage point of each group member results in a more complete and comprehensive description of the elephant (Streubert and Carpenter, 1999). In the context of the present investigation, triangulation was expected to contribute 'an additional piece of the puzzle' (Shih, 1998, p. 633). Furthermore, Cutcliffe and McKenna (1999) argue that if a triangulated approach is used in conjunction with other attempts to establish credibility then the researcher has made a thorough attempt to address issues of representativeness and credibility of their qualitative research findings.

TRUSTWORTHINESS

While some have argued that qualitative research is less rigorous than quantitative work (Conway, 1998), qualitative researchers would disagree (Grbich, 1999). According to Guba and Lincoln (1989), 'trustworthiness' criteria in qualitative research set out to do what 'rigour' criteria have done in the quantitative paradigm. Internal validity, external validity, reliability and objectivity criteria are perfectly reasonable and appropriate in logical positivism contexts since they are 'grounded in the ontological and epistemological framework of that paradigm' (Guba and Lincoln, 1989, p. 235). Conversely, the parallel criteria – credibility, dependability, confirmability and transferability – are more appropriate in qualitative research. The ultimate goal of trustworthiness in qualitative research is to represent accurately study participants' experiences.

To ensure the trustworthiness of the present study, a number of strategies were employed as recommended by Hamilton *et al.* (1977), Guba and Lincoln (1989) and Robson (1993). It is argued that there has been a shift in focus in qualitative research in that 'it is important to establish a match between the constructed realities of respondents and those realities as represented by the evaluator' (Guba and Lincoln, 1989, p. 236). By doing so, findings can be judged as credible. The techniques recommended to increase the likelihood of this, and adopted in the present investigation, include 'prolonged engagement', 'persistent observation' and 'member checks' (Guba and Lincoln, 1989). These measures were incorporated into the study by maintaining contact with participants in each Case Site over an 18-month duration, the recording of supervision sessions and collection of CS session records and critical incident journals over a 12- to 18-month duration and returning to participants to discuss data analysis. Further, multiple triangulation, as detailed above, was adopted.

Additionally, my academic supervisors conducted an independent analysis of a sample of the interview and audio-recording transcripts using Heron's (1989) analytic framework. Similarly, I requested my academic supervisors to develop their own categorisations from the qualitative data – interview transcripts, CS session records, critical incident journals and audio-recordings using 'thematic analysis'. Finally, I returned to participants and asked them to comment on the transcripts, how their quotes 'fitted' with the analytic framework and the categorisation of the themes generated from the thematic analysis. These strategies are considered to have enhanced the credibility of these data.

Guba and Lincoln (1989, p. 242) write: 'The constructivist paradigm's assurances of integrity of the findings are rooted in the data themselves.' The interview transcripts, session documents, CS session records, critical incident journals and audio-recordings of supervision are available in order to confirm that findings are rooted in the data and have not been developed by other means.

In qualitative research, the transferability of findings depends to some extent upon the nature of the study's sample and upon the context of the study. The term 'transferability' corresponds approximately to the notion of generalisability in quantitative research (Guba and Lincoln, 1989). I endeavoured to provide a 'thick', contextually relevant description of clinical CS as used by mental health nurses in a Primary Care Trust. Team descriptions (the learning milieu), documents relevant to how CS has been progressed in the Trust (instructional system) and the other data derived from this investigation contributed to this account. This detailed and extensive description will enable potential users of the research to decide how 'transferable' are the findings of this study. Accordingly, Guba and Lincoln (1989, p. 241) argue that 'the burden of proof for claimed transferability is on the receiver', rather than the researcher. Morse (1999) proposes that the knowledge gained from the theory should fit all scenarios that may be identified in the larger population. Furthermore, she stresses: 'the theory is also applicable to all similar situations, questions, and problems, regardless of the comparability of the demographic composition of the groups' (Morse, 1999, p. 5).

DATA ANALYSIS

The exploration of interpersonal interactions was an important focus of this investigation. Consequently, a number of analytic strategies that make use of different theories of interpersonal exchanges were considered for the analysis of the semi-structured in-depth interviews and audio-recordings of supervision (Chapter 3). Chapter 4 provided further consideration and discussion on these analytic frameworks.

It was felt that 'thematic content analysis' as described by Burnard (1991) could be useful for the analysis of all data generated in the current study. However, as noted in Chapter 3, the term 'thematic analysis' was adopted for this thesis. Thematic analysis is considered an appropriate method when the data have been derived from semi-structured, open-ended interviews and has been audio-recorded and transcribed in full. When using thematic analysis, the aim is to produce a detailed and systematic recording of the themes and issues addressed during the interviews together under a reasonably exhaustive category system (Burnard, 1991). In the present study, thematic analysis was used to analyse data derived from semi-structured interviews, audio-recordings of supervision sessions, critical incident journals and CS session records. Thus, all the study's data were analysed using thematic analysis (Burnard, 1991). This was done by reading and re-reading the transcripts and using Microsoft Word.

Burnard's (1991) 'thematic content analysis' has been used extensively in nursing research to analyse semi-structured and unstructured interview data. Burnard (1991) describes 14 stages for his thematic analysis method. These are described in the context of the present study.

Stage 1 Notes were made following the semi-structured interview using a contact summary sheet. I also wrote memos at various points during the research project. Memos can develop the researcher's ideas on how to categorise the data, assist in theorising about emerging themes and be a useful memory jogger (Burnard, 1991).

Stage 2 The transcripts were read through and notes were made on general themes within the transcripts. Burnard (1991, p. 462) suggests that the aim here is 'to become immersed in the data'. Ultimately, I wanted to get an appreciation of participants' perspectives on CS.

Stage 3 Transcripts were read through a second time and as many headings as necessary were written down so that all aspects of the content were described. Categories were generated freely at this stage. According to Burnard (1991), the 'category system' should account for most of the data.

Stage 4 The list of categories was reviewed and these were grouped together under higher-order headings. Here, the intention was to collapse similar categories into broader categories.

Stage 5 This new list of categories and subheadings was worked through and repetitious headings were removed to produce a final list.

Stage 6 Burnard (1991, p. 463) advises: 'two colleagues are invited to generate category systems independently without seeing the researcher's list'. In the present study, my three academic supervisors generated separate category systems. These were discussed and adjustments were made as necessary.

Stage 7 The transcripts were reviewed again alongside the final list of categories and subheadings to establish the degree to which the categories covered all aspects of the data.

Stage 8   Each transcript was worked through with the list of categories and subheadings and 'coded' according to the list of category headings.

Stage 9   Each coded section was 'cut' out of the transcript and collected together according to the category it belonged using Microsoft Word 2000's 'cut and paste'. For reference purposes, Burnard (1991) argues that it is important to keep a 'whole' transcript for each data source.

Stage 10   The cut-out sections were 'copied' onto sheets headed up with category headings and subheadings.

Stage 11   Selected participants were asked to check the appropriateness of their quotations in the various categories. This allows for a check on the trustworthiness/credibility of the categorising process.

Stage 12   All sections were filed together for direct reference when writing up the findings. As mentioned previously, copies of the complete transcripts and the original recordings were kept at hand during the writing-up stage. Thus, if there was any confusion during this stage, I could refer to the original transcript or recording.

Stage 13   Burnard (1991) describes this as the writing-up stage.

Stage 14   According to Burnard (1991), the researcher must decide how he or she is going to link the data examples and commentary to the existing literature. He offers two options. First, findings and discussion can be written up as two distinct sections. Second, findings can be written up alongside reference to current literature. A combination of these was used in the present study.

As stated previously, a number of analytic strategies that drew upon different theories of interpersonal exchanges were considered (Chapter 4). As argued in Chapter 4, Heron's framework was considered a useful analytic tool for the present study. Moreover, by undertaking a secondary analysis, the trustworthiness of the emerging categories was secured. Kimchi *et al.* (1991) argue that by comparing results of data analysed using differing qualitative analysis techniques enables researchers to note similar patterns and therefore verify findings. Despite the fact that secondary analysis proved extremely time-consuming, challenging and complicated, Heron's framework was used to analyse a proportion of the data, the interview transcripts and supervisors' contribution from the audio-recordings of supervision sessions. The supervisees' contribution was captured from Burnard's (1991) thematic content analysis. Together, this analysis revealed supervisor–supervisee interactions and their influence on session content.

ETHICAL CONSIDERATIONS

Ethical considerations for this study emerged during the initial planning stages. A key aspect of this study was concerned with the supervisory relationship and specifically the reciprocal exchanges between clinical supervisor and supervisee during their supervision sessions. Asking clinical supervisors and supervisees to express their views on this relationship was thought to be potentially intrusive. The researcher, in acknowledging expectations of confidentiality in CS and the nature of issues often discussed, was aware of possibly influencing these discussions. Many clinicians use the supervisory process to reflect on clinical practice, and specifically to improve areas of practice. Exposing this normally private discussion and any likely sensitive information required careful ethical consideration. Further, I had to consider the possible consequences following this content being exposed. As Patton (1990) acknowledges, the process of being interviewed may leave the interviewee more aware of things about themselves than they did prior to the interview. Moreover, interviewees may divulge more about themselves during an interview than they intended.

Several strategies were implemented to address these concerns and also provide protection to potential research participants. Four ethical principles as outlined by the Royal College of Nursing (RCN, 1998) – beneficence, nonmaleficence, respect for autonomy and justice – were adopted and provided a guide to the ethical approach in this study. Collectively, these broad concepts address the issues highlighted by Hayter:

> If human rights are to be adequately protected attention must be given to the rights of informed consent, privacy, confidentiality – anonymity of data, protection from harm, and the right to refuse or withdraw from participation without recrimination. (Hayter, 1979, p. 109)

The principle of beneficence holds that we should try and do good (RCN, 1998). While this study did not aim to improve patient care directly, the improvement of patient care has been an alleged benefit of CS (Bishop, 1994; Goorapah, 1997) and a much-sought-after outcome (Wray et al., 1998; Bassett, 2000). Although this potential for improvement may not be immediate, it is anticipated that findings emerging from the present study may have some influence on the capacity of CS to improve patient care over time. Furthermore, by having an aspect of this study focus on identifying the facilitative and constraining factors that influence the scope of CS, I aimed to illuminate the effective delivery of individual CS for mental health nurses. The study's findings may also be relevant to nurses working in other settings, for example general surgical/medical areas, palliative care and intensive care. The results of the current study may increase existing knowledge and understanding of CS and may make a contribution to shaping the CS practices of counsellors, psychologists and other professional groups. This knowledge will be appropriately disseminated in order to help develop the practice of CS in the future.

Participants may have benefited from their direct involvement in this investigation. They may have gained from having the opportunity to express their views on the CS they received and by reflecting on the supervisory process during the in-depth interviews. Participants may also have gained satisfaction from participating in the study and knowing their contribution will possibly influence improvements to the local provision of supervision.

The principle of non-maleficence holds that no harm will come to research participants as a direct result of their involvement (RCN, 1998). All participants were reassured that there would be no health risk as a result of participating in this study. As highlighted previously, informants can often feel they have disclosed too much. My experience as a mental health nurse, an accredited cognitive psychotherapist and being sensitive to others helped me to gauge how far to probe particular issues with individuals. Indeed, the interview guide had been developed with this concern in mind. As a result, questions were organised in a gradual way starting with less provocative issues and progressing to sensitive concerns. Moreover, during the interview, I frequently inquired if participants were comfortable enough to continue talking about particular aspects of their supervisory experience.

The data-collection methods had been chosen for their ability to generate rich data. More importantly, they were thought to cause minimal disruption to participants' everyday work practices. For example, session documents were already completed by some participants and therefore did not demand additional time. For participants' convenience, interviews were conducted at their preferred location. No demands were made on participants to engage in additional supervision sessions – I was interested to learn about the supervision in which they were already engaged. Thus, clinical supervisors and supervisees were asked to audio-record their routine sessions.

The ability to make free choices about oneself and one's life is at the centre of the principle of autonomy (Brink and Wood, 1994; RCN, 1998). In acknowledging this principle, I endeavoured to ensure that all participants were given free and informed consent to take part in research. First and foremost, all participants were invited into the study on a voluntary basis. However, before this could happen, each participant required information in order for him or her to give informed consent. Furthermore, participants were informed that they could withdraw from the study at any time without adverse consequences to themselves (Christman and Johnson, 1981).

Prior to this consent being requested, each participant was provided with an explanation of the major aspects of the study and the extent of their involvement. It was necessary to develop a specific consent form for each of the various groups of participants. That is, the level of involvement by the PSMs was quite different from that of the clinical supervisors' and supervisees'; the information required by them to make an informed consent varied.

Information, as recommended by Smith (1992) and RCN (1998), was shared with participants. Informed consent detailing the aims of the study, purpose of the research, identifying the researcher, academic supervisors, educational institution, identifying where the study would take place, how individuals were selected and what participation would involve was sought from participants. However, as suggested previously, the exact content did vary and was dependent on the participants' expected involvement in the study.

Before progressing with the data collection at each site, I met with each participant and provided an explanation of the study and confirmed his or her informed consent. However, I met with supervision pairs (clinical supervisor and supervisee) to obtain their joint consent prior to audio-recording sessions. Each participant was given his or her own copy of the consent form. As usual and necessary in qualitative research, I re-negotiate this consent on an ongoing basis throughout the study. Lastly, during preparation for the in-depth interview, a further explanation of the study was offered.

Furthermore, during the ongoing research process, other strategies aiming to maintain ethical soundness (Robson, 1993) were adopted. For example, negotiating with participants regarding the description/interpretation of their account made by the researcher, returning to participants and seeking their validation of the quotations and their fit with the category within which they are found and obtaining explicit authorisation before using particular quotations.

Confidentiality and anonymity were assured. All participants were given a pseudonym. However, since there was only one PSM and TL for each team (learning milieu), their anonymity, from an organisational perspective, could have been threatened. This was highlighted when seeking their informed consent at the outset and re-negotiated throughout the study. All interviews were conducted in private surroundings. Participants' names were not used on any of the study's material except consent forms and on a master list of participants' names and their pseudonym. These were stored within a locked filing cabinet within the researcher's office at work and home. Only the researcher has had access to this information. All research material made available to the researcher's academic supervisors was coded or used a pseudonym. Participants were advised that information obtained during the study might be submitted to a professional journal for publication or used for a conference paper. However, their names would not be associated with any aspect of such a publication. The stipulations contained within the Data Protection Act 1998 were adhered to.

ETHICAL APPROVAL AND ACCESS TO PARTICIPANTS

The research proposal was discussed with the Director of the Mental Health Service and access to the MHD was given. Following an application to the Department of Nursing and Community Health's Ethics Committee, Glasgow Caledonian University and the Primary Care Trust's Clinical Effectiveness Committee, ethical approval was granted for the study to be carried out. The research proposal was approved without amendment. While not a requirement for ethical approval, the proposal was also submitted to the Primary Care Trust's Ethics Committee and the relevant Health Board's Ethics Committee for information.

CONCLUSION

This chapter has described the study's design and methods chosen in order to address the research questions central to the present study. In order to provide clarity of the learning milieux, a thorough description of each Case Site was presented. Key issues relevant to two aspects of the instructional system preceded a presentation of how the data-collection techniques were adopted. Before illustrating findings for the main study, experience from the pilot study and how it influenced the investigation thereafter is described in the following chapter.

6 Pilot Study

INTRODUCTION

It was acknowledged (Chapter 2) that research on the interpersonal transactions integral to the supervisory experience is not without its difficulties. In consideration of possible reluctance from participants to engage in certain aspects of the data-collection methods as described by Malin (2000), I wanted to determine if the proposed study was feasible. The aims of the pilot study were:

- to determine if the proposed study was feasible (participants, access, time);
- to identify potential problems with the components of the research design;
- to help develop and refine data-collection methods;
- to determine if the sampling strategy was appropriate and realistic;
- to examine the trustworthiness of the data-generating techniques and the emerging data;
- to refine the data-analysis plan and to clarify if the emerging data could be usefully analysed using Heron's analytic framework;
- to increase the researcher's knowledge and understanding of Heron's analytic framework;
- to provide experience with all aspects of the study including participants, setting, data-collection techniques, recording equipment and data analysis.

This chapter provides a description of the pilot study and the experiences and insights gained from this process.

LOCATION, PARTICIPANTS AND ACCESS

Every effort was made to ensure participants in the pilot study were as similar to those who would be invited into the main study. Purposive sampling (Chinn, 1986; Munhall and Oiler, 1986) was used to invite those participants from an adult CMHT within the MHD of the Trust. A description of how access to the research site was sought and the process of ethical approval are described in the previous chapter. Access to the team was negotiated with the relevant PSM and TL.

CASE SITE DESCRIPTION

The team was one of six adult CMHTs. The main aims of the team were to provide assessment, treatment, continuing care and support in the community to people with serious and enduring mental health problems, and to others with less serious problems, with early intervention aimed at promoting and maintaining the mental health of individuals and their families and/or carers. The team was multi-disciplinary and had clinicians from nursing, psychiatry, clinical psychology, occupational therapy and social work. A team secretary, medical secretary and clerical officer provided clerical support. The TL had a nursing background.

STAFF COMPLEMENT FOR PILOT STUDY SITE

TL (H grade)	Steve
CN (G grade)	Frank and Emily
SN (E grade)	Jennifer and Bonnie
Consultant psychiatrist	(4 sessions)
Clinical psychologist	(5 sessions)
Occupational therapist	(10 sessions)
Social worker	(5 sessions)
Administrative staff	(4)

PARTICIPANTS AND THEIR TEAM ROLE

The majority of qualified nursing staff and relevant managers, which included Allan (PSM), Steve (TL), Frank and Emily (CNs) and Jennifer and Bonnie (SNs), agreed to participate in the study (Figure 6.1). At the time of the study, Allan and Steve each had more than 20 years' experience working in mental health; Frank, Emily, Jennifer and Bonnie had worked in mental health nursing for between ten and 15 years. Steve had completed a diploma in community psychiatric nursing. Frank had completed a short course on counselling.

On average, the SNs each had a caseload of 35 patients. Caseload mix was 60% enduring needs and 40% brief needs, though some nurses' caseload mix diverged from this. General practices all had a nominated liaison nurse who accepted and followed up the majority of referrals. Provision was made for this clinical work to be spread amongst other nurses if any particular practice referred an unduly large number of patients. One nurse was designated each day to respond to urgent calls. Allocation of student nurses was done on a rotational basis, and all qualified nurses were preceptors.

This team had no team protocol, policy document or written account of their supervisory format. The TL made available the CS discussion paper developed within the Trust (Chapter 5). In the absence of any documentation, participants agreed to use the session record developed for the purposes of the study.

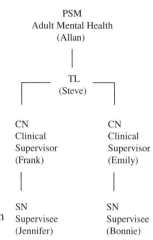

Figure 6.1 Case Sites, participants and their function for the pilot study.

DATA-COLLECTION METHODS

INTERVIEW

All participants agreed to the semi-structured in-depth interview. Conducting these interviews provided the opportunity of using each of the interview schedules. The interview generated important qualitative data, and the multi-perspective on CS was helpful in contributing to generating a complete and comprehensive data set. It helped to prevent a peculiar and perhaps biased perception of CS from emerging. Analysis of the data derived from interviews with Allan, Steve, Frank, Emily and Jennifer was conducted.

At the completion of the interview, all of the participants declined when asked if they had anything further to add. On the contrary, they commented on the comprehensiveness of the questions and the variety of issues covered. No suggestions were offered for additional topics. All participants thought that their individual experience of CS had been captured with the questions in the interview schedule.

CLINICAL SUPERVISION SESSION RECORD

Jennifer and Bonnie (supervisees) completed the CS session record and commented that sections proved useful in providing relevant data.

CRITICAL INCIDENT JOURNAL

Jennifer and Bonnie completed one entry of their critical incident journal. These examples gave further information on how supervision was used, issues relating to the supervisory relationship (conflict) and both helpful and unhelpful supervisor behaviours.

AUDIO-RECORDING OF CLINICAL SUPERVISION

Both supervision pairs (Frank and Jennifer, Emily and Bonnie) provided one audio-recording of a supervision session. No concerns were expressed regarding the recording equipment. Participants found the recording equipment easy to use and, perhaps more importantly, not intrusive when the supervision session was being recorded. The audio-recording with Frank and Jennifer was transcribed and analysed.

Participants' views on these data-collection methods were also sought; no negative feedback was offered.

DATA ANALYSIS

The pilot study provided an opportunity for me to become more familiar with Heron's (1989) framework and helped to increase my knowledge and understanding of the various categories. Furthermore, it helped to determine whether the framework was appropriate for the analysis of the interview transcripts and audio-recordings of supervision sessions.

In the first analysis of transcripts from in-depth interviews with Allan, Steve, Frank and Jennifer, and a transcript of an audio-recording of a supervision session with Frank and Jennifer, Heron's framework was used as a conceptual template. Once all transcripts had been analysed, excerpts of these were sent to each member of the academic supervisory team asking them to conduct an independent analysis of the transcripts using Heron's framework. This exercise was beneficial, and generally these independent analyses conflated with each other. Differences were slight and the result of the academic supervisory team not having access to the audio-recording of the supervision session while analysing that particular transcript. Hearing how supervisor and supervisee interacted, particularly the paralinguistic aspects of their speech acts, influenced how transcripts were analysed.

Of more concern was the fact that large quantities of each of the transcripts were not absorbed by any of the categories. Using the framework as a conceptual framework resulted in copious amounts of unusable data. Heron's framework is focused on behaviours of the helper. Consequently, the content of supervision or, indeed, the supervisee's contribution to the supervision session was not captured. Similarly, changes resulting from CS did not emerge when using Heron's framework.

Subsequently, a further analysis was carried out using a transcript of the interview with Emily (clinical supervisor). This transcript was analysed using open thematic analysis as described by Burnard (1991). All members of the academic supervisory team were given excerpts of the transcript and, following this consultation, a final list of categories was developed. The following categories emerged:

- stimulus for the focus of supervision;
- structure of supervision;
- content of supervision session;
- supervisor interventions;
- supervisee contribution;
- obstacles to supervision;
- potential effects/outcomes from supervision.

The audio-recording of the supervision session with Frank and Jennifer was then analysed using the seven categories. My academic supervisors conducted an independent analysis of this transcript. Thereafter, an open thematic analysis (Burnard, 1991) was conducted on the interview transcripts from Allan, Steve, Frank and Jennifer, session records and critical incident journal entries. Finally, an additional analysis of data from the audio-recording of the supervision session (Frank and Jennifer) was carried out using Heron's (1989) analytic framework. The triangulated analysis of the transcript from the CS session, involving Frank and Jennifer, is illustrated in the following section.

ANALYSIS OF AN AUDIO-RECORDING OF A SUPERVISION SESSION

This section provides part of the detailed analysis of a CS session that was audio-recorded and transcribed verbatim. Triangulation analysis using thematic analysis (Burnard, 1991) and Heron's (1989) analytic framework was conducted. In the following sections, I will present some of the interpersonal processes and, in particular, the delivery of supervisor interventions during a supervision session.

Stimuli for the focus of supervision

Throughout the session, the pace and the time spent on specific issues were directed largely by the clinical supervisor. At the start of the session, Frank implied 'progress' as the stimulus for focusing on feedback regarding cases discussed during previous sessions.

> Just to feed back on the last supervision in the record and see if there is any progress or how have things been in relation to particular clients, the role of the psychologists in one particular client.
>
> (Frank, audio-recording, 20/10/98, p. 1)

In response, Jennifer gave a detailed update on the 'progress' of two previously discussed cases that concerned referring a client on to another service
and maintaining contact with a client while awaiting assessment from another
service. In addition to giving some insight into what stimulated the content of
the supervision sessions, Frank's request for feedback on previously discussed
cases demonstrated the potential for illuminating changes in Jennifer's practice over time.

From Jennifer's perspective, the stimuli for focus during this session were
her uncertainty in working with three particular clients and her concerns
regarding the introduction of a risk-assessment procedure. Suicide risk was a
common theme in each of these issues. While Jennifer did not make a direct
request for help with this, her anxieties were demonstrated in the presentation of her clinical work and the recurrent theme of suicide risk in the cases
discussed during this session.

> She took a fairly serious overdose a year or so ago. Fairly impulsive like, when
> she was down. I think she had been in hospital and was out on pass, had gone out
> and had taken the tablets. So obviously there are concerns as to her kind of
> vulnerability.
> (Jennifer, audio-recording, 20/10/98, p. 6)

> There are, there is always, not always, but on several occasions there's been fleet-
> ing thoughts of . . . of suicide or self-harm . . . obviously it's putting into a care
> package, you know, how she really is, you know, there is the kind of fleeting
> thoughts of suicide but no serious plan or intent to act on those.
> (Jennifer, audio-recording, 20/10/98, p. 8)

> I think what was concerning myself and other staff members was the fact that
> there's a part in the form, 'Do you or do you not think that the client is at risk',
> you know?
> (Jennifer, audio-recording, 20/10/98, p. 16)

Structure

The session took place at a clinic outwith of the team base and lasted 45
minutes. There was a balance between supervisor- and supervisee-generated
items for discussion. However, as identified earlier and to be developed later,
the clinical supervisor directed the session throughout.

Content

Both the clinical supervisor and the supervisee generated items for this
session. From Frank's perspective, this included feedback on previously
discussed cases, reducing Jennifer's caseload, seeking an update on a
client's depot medication and seeking feedback on a recently introduced

'pre-allocation of new referrals' procedure. In addition to responding to these items, the supervisee focused on aspects of her clinical work. Jennifer engaged in discussion concerning the monitoring of a client's mental health and their vulnerability to further suicide attempts, devising a care plan for a 'suicide risk' client, reviewing a client's depot medication and highlighting her concerns with the pilot project of a risk-assessment procedure.

The 'content' of the session supports findings from previous research using self-report methods. White *et al.* (1998) report that participants in the large-scale multi-site evaluation study used CS to discuss organisational and management issues, clinical casework, professional development, educational support, confidence building, interpersonal problems and personal matters. However, the influence of supervisor interventions on the priority and extent of discussion became clearer when supervisor interventions were illuminated.

Supervisor interventions

This broad category has several subthemes:

- exploring the supervisee's work;
- reflecting back;
- taking the lead;
- suggesting an option;
- being supportive;
- giving information.

In this section, the potential of analysis triangulation using Burnard's (1991) thematic analysis and Heron's (1989) analytic framework will be illustrated. Findings relating to exploring the supervisee's work, taking the lead, suggesting an option and giving feedback will be presented. The most common strategy used by the clinical supervisor in this session was exploring the supervisee's work.

Exploring the supervisee's work

> Well, how do you think she'll cope if you're not there; how do you think you know if you aren't around until psychology kicks in; how do you think that will affect her?
>
> (Frank, audio-recording, 20/10/98, p. 3)

However, the majority of the information-gathering questions asked by the clinical supervisor were delivered as closed questions, thus limiting the response and exploration of the supervisee.

> Would she consider the () centre?
>
> (Frank, audio-recording, 20/10/98, p. 7)

Taking the lead

Despite there being a balance between supervisor and supervisee items on the agenda, the clinical supervisor controlled the time and level of discussion on particular items.

> Moving on, another client requiring treatment from psychology, limited input until psychology can taken her on?
> (Frank, audio-recording, 20/10/98, p. 2)

Suggesting an option

On a few occasions, the clinical supervisor would make a suggestion on how the supervisee might proceed with some of her clinical work. In the following example, Frank suggested some issues for Jennifer to discuss with the client.

> And they give work placements via () as well, which is an option. I think I'd put these things to her, you know, as maybe an idea.
> (Frank, audio-recording, 20/10/98, p. 8)

Giving information

A frequently reported expectation of CS is the development of professional skills (Butterworth and Faugier, 1992; DoH, 1993; UKCC, 1996; Cutcliffe and Burns, 1998; Lowry, 1998; Kelly *et al.*, 2001). One might assume, therefore, that supervisor interventions might focus on this development for the supervisee. Interestingly, although not used often in this session, information-giving by the supervisor focused on supervisor-generated items for the session concerning team-policy issues rather than the development of specific clinical skills.

> There's a meeting on Wednesday to discuss it.
> (Frank, audio-recording, 20/10/98, p. 15)

Catalytic interventions

When using Heron's (1989) framework to analyse the supervision transcript, the most frequently used category of intervention was catalytic. According to Heron (1989), a catalytic intervention is one that promotes self-discovery, self-directed living, learning and problem-solving in the client. In this session, specific catalytic interventions included open questions, closed questions, checking for understanding and paraphrasing. The following example is typical of the closed questions Frank would ask.

> So () is quite happy to wait?
> (Frank, audio-recording, 20/10/98, p. 2)

There are obvious similarities between the subcategories from the thematic analysis category 'supervisor interventions' – exploring an issue and reflecting back – and the catalytic category from Heron's analytic framework. Heron (1989, p. 101) states: 'In general, open questions tend to be more catalytic than closed questions simply because they give more scope for self-directed exploration and discovery.'

In this session the use of open questions was limited. Conversely, there was an abundant reliance on closed questions, perhaps constraining the supervisee's opportunity for discovery.

Prescriptive interventions

Heron (1989, p. 30) asserts: 'Prescriptive interventions seek to influence and direct the behaviour of the client especially, though not exclusively, behaviour that is outside or beyond the practitioner–client interaction.' Prescriptive interventions were delivered throughout the session and are captured as 'taking the lead' and 'suggesting an option' from the thematic analysis.

> And they give work placements as well, which is an option. I think I'd put these things to her, you know, as maybe an idea.
> (Frank, audio-recording, 20/10/98, p. 8)

Informative interventions

Some of the supervisor interventions that fall within the thematic analysis category 'giving information' fit with Heron's (1989) informative category. As previously highlighted, informative interventions related mostly to the sharing of team-policy issues and were derived from the clinical supervisor's agenda. Although undoubtedly relevant to this supervisee's practice, such organisationally focused information-giving may be at odds with progressing clinical practice and ultimately dilute the potential for the supervisee's professional development. In the following example, Frank informed Jennifer of a team meeting regarding a new method for the allocation of referrals.

> There's a meeting on Wednesday to discuss it.
> (Frank, audio-recording, 20/10/98, p. 15)

Supportive interventions

Heron (1989, p. 120) explains: 'Supportive interventions affirm the worth and value of the person, of their qualities, attitudes of mind, actions, artefacts and creations.' In the example that follows, Frank appeared to affirm Jennifer's experience in working with this client. Jennifer's belief that the client 'jumps from pillar to post, discussing a lot of topics' was validated. The confirmation of nursing actions has been reported as an important benefit of group supervision (Palsson *et al.*, 1994; Begat *et al.*, 1997; Arvidsson *et al.*, 2000). In these studies, the effect of confirmation appeared to develop from discussions between other supervisees. However, from the pilot study, an example of how Frank confirmed Jennifer's thoughts was illuminated.

> Because, as you say, her presentation just jumps from pillar to post, discussing a lot of topics.
> (Frank, audio-recording, 20/10/98, p. 10)

Degenerate interventions

In this session, Frank did not offer any interventions that could be classified as cathartic or confronting. Instead, he delivered catalytic, prescriptive, informative and supportive interventions. However, this is not to say that the opportunity for incorporating these interventions did not arise during the session. An important contribution of Heron's framework is the recognition given to unhelpful interventions. This aspect of the framework gives consideration to what is not done during CS as well as to those interventions delivered that may be classified as unhelpful.

In this session, from the supervisee's perspective, an issue for the agenda, though not made explicit, was concerned with her uncertainty and anxiety regarding working with clients expressing suicidal ideation. Jennifer's unease went unnoticed by Frank. Towards the end of the session, the supervisee attempted to return to this issue by making reference to a risk-assessment tool that was being piloted in the team. Again, Frank made no acknowledgement of this unease. Instead, he emphasised the supervisee's unfamiliarity with the forms being used during the pilot risk assessment.

> This is it; it's a new thing 'pilot form'; it's a new thing.
> (Frank, audio-recording, 20/10/98, p. 17)

This may be interpreted as a cathartic degenerate intervention and specifically 'not giving permission' (Heron, 1989, p. 158). Bowles and Young (1999, p. 960) make the claim that 'clinical supervision has been uncritically accepted as being good for every nurse and likely to be of equal good for every nurse'. There has been an absence of attention on unhelpful aspects of CS in the nursing literature. Following analysis of data from the pilot study, an example of a degenerate intervention emerged.

When using Heron's framework to analyse supervisor verbal transactions, examples of catalytic, prescriptive, informative and supportive interventions became evident. There was an absence of cathartic and confronting interventions. This conflates with findings from previous work where nurses reported being least skilled in using cathartic and confronting interventions (Burnard and Morrison, 1988, 1991; Morrison and Burnard, 1989).

It is important to emphasise that this interpretation was derived from an audio-recording of one session. Rather than try to convince the reader that this interpretation is definitive, the pilot study has highlighted the potential of using Heron's framework as an additional analytic template with which to secure the comprehensiveness of the data. In the main study, the longitudinal nature of the study's design was expected to enhance the credibility of these data.

The supervisee's contribution

Evident from this session was the supervisee's contribution to the discussion. This included having specific items for the supervision agenda, all of which had a clinical focus and, as in the following example, were asking for guidance.

> I think by a letter. I'll send her a letter just asking if she needs any kind of support in the interim between now and psychology being involved. Do you think that's appropriate?
>
> (Jennifer, audio-recording, 20/10/98, p. 2)

Obstacles to supervision

As previously mentioned, the clinical supervisor directed much of the discussion during this session. In particular, the supervisor controlled the level of discussion for each of the items by prompting progression to another item. This may have constrained the supervisee's exploration of particular issues. The amount of time available to discuss the items on their agenda may have been a stimulus for this control. A possible result of this was that the clinical supervisor did not 'hear' the supervisee's anxieties concerning suicide risk.

Potential changes resulting from clinical supervision

From the transcript of this session and as previously highlighted, there is the potential to follow up changes in the supervisee's practice. The discussions, which take place during CS, may have some relevance to this progression. Issues from this session that may have been followed up include monitoring the client's mental health, distraction activities for a client, development of a problem list for a client, review of a client's depot medication, use of the risk-assessment tool to assess suicide risk, reducing caseload size and the experience of the 'pre-allocation of new referrals' procedure.

CONCLUSION

This chapter has suggested that participants' enthusiasm for CS generally promoted their willingness to engage in the pilot study. The participants reported that they recognised the potential for this focus of study and appreciated the opportunity to share their experiences. Participants expressed gratitude at having the opportunity to reflect on their engagement in CS. No concerns were raised regarding the time needed to complete the CS session record or the critical incident journal. Participants felt at ease in having a supervision session audio-recorded and mentioned that they soon forgot about the recording equipment. No problems were identified with using the recording equipment.

The evaluation approach known as illuminative evaluation was considered appropriate and relevant to investigating the questions central to the main study listed in Chapter 3. Moreover, the triangulation methodology was considered appropriate in providing a rich and comprehensive interpretation of the changes resulting from CS. Conceptualising a team as a Case Site and the learning milieu was useful in exploring the supervisory process and the influence of particular supervision interventions on this.

The data-generating methods produced a wealth of qualitative data. Following the pilot study, it was concluded that these methods were suitable for exploring areas of conceptual interest for the main study. A purposive sampling strategy was felt suitable for enabling those informants who had the necessary experience with CS to be engaged in the main study.

Following a detailed analysis of the pilot study's data, it was decided that all data in the main study would be analysed using Burnard's (1991) thematic analysis. A secondary analysis of the interview transcripts and audio-recordings of CS sessions using Heron's (1989) framework would also be conducted. The pilot study helped to increase my appreciation and understanding of these analytic methods.

7 Report of Findings and Discussion

INTRODUCTION

Chapters 7, 8 and 9 of my PhD thesis (Sloan, 2004) present findings relating to Case Site One, Two and Three respectively. In each of these chapters, some aspects of the findings were illustrated by selective reference to the literature. It was noted that some categories from the open thematic analysis were common across all three sites, but no overall integration of the study's findings had been undertaken in those chapters.

In this chapter, a comprehensive discussion of findings across all three sites and their relevance to current literature will be provided. The study objectives, which were described in Chapter 3, and the related findings will be used as a basis for the discussion. Conclusions will be drawn from the overall findings. Core and sub-categories will be placed in single quotation marks.

OBJECTIVES OF THE STUDY

The objectives of the study were stated in Chapter 3. These were to:

1. identify the uses of individual CS made by mental health nurses working in an NHS Primary Care Trust;
2. explore and describe supervisees' experiences of individual CS;
3. describe how the organisational provision of CS influences the supervisory process;
4. analyse the interactions between the supervisor and supervisee during supervision;
5. explore how these interactions influence the content of supervision;
6. illuminate the changes resulting from supervision, as reported by participants.

OBJECTIVE 1

To identify the uses of individual CS made by mental health nurses working in an NHS Primary Care Trust.

Triangulating various data-collection methods illuminated the uses of CS. The data-collection methods included individual in-depth interviews with all participants, audio-recording of supervision sessions involving the clinical supervisor and supervisee, CS session records and critical incident journals that were maintained by supervisees.

CS appeared to have a broad scope in the setting for this investigation. A theme common to all three teams concerned CS being used for the discussion of issues deemed important by the clinical supervisor. Clinical supervisors, having a line-management role over supervisees, appeared to have a strong influence over managerial issues taking precedence. Furthermore, CS appeared to have strong associations with counselling and therapy and, in two teams, was thought to have therapeutic intentions and subsequent therapeutic outcome. Clinical and, specifically, client-related issues did feature during CS, but discussions were focused on managing the caseload rather than exploring the complexity of these issues. Lastly, there appeared to be an understanding in all three teams that anything and everything could be taken to supervision.

Managerial agendas

While Darley (2001) and others support the view that CS can be provided by a manager, Cutcliffe (2000a) suggests that managerial supervision should run parallel to, not concomitant with, CS. The UK nursing literature highlights considerable support for the management-led model for the delivery of CS and that it is common for supervisory arrangements to be hierarchical (White *et al.*, 1998; Cutcliffe, 2000a). Wolsey and Leach (1997), for example, argue that CS develops practitioners' talents in preparation for their next post. They debate the necessity to demonstrate that supervision 'contributes to improving quality, levels of service, speed of service delivery and reduced costs' (Wolsey and Leach, 1997, p. 26).

Research conducted by Scanlon and Weir (1997), Kipping (1998), Sloan (1999), Duncan-Grant (2000a) and Kelly *et al.* (2001) in mental health nursing has highlighted a similar trend. A number of participants in Scanlon and Weir's (1997) study were suspicious and lacked trust when they were supervised by their immediate manager. In a study conducted in Scotland investigating CS in community mental health nursing, Sloan (1999) found that as a result of the supervisor also having a managerial role management issues were taken to a CS session. A similar emphasis was apparent in Kelly *et al.*'s (2001) survey of community mental health nurses' perceptions of CS in Northern Ireland.

Duncan-Grant (2000a) reports that the supervisor for participants in his investigation were almost exclusively their line manager. Senior managers had good reason to organise CS in this way. From their perspective, senior staff supervising subordinates facilitated the 'passing on of wisdom' by experienced to less experienced staff, and for supervisees to receive 'good advice' and 'check out their actions' (Duncan-Grant, 2000a, p. 400). Not surprisingly, senior staff regarded staff surveillance as an explicit function of CS. Concerns such as these, according to Yegdich (1999b), primarily belong to managerial supervision. More importantly, she argues that CS could only function on a foundation of managerial supervision and staff welfare, support and education.

Participants from all teams in the current study reported that there were no separate meetings with line managers for managerial supervision. Performance appraisals, professional development planning, communicating annual leave and off-duty, and discussion about staff relations, were all incorporated into CS. Managerial agendas overshadowed clinical issues.

CS appeared to be endorsed as a risk-management strategy and categories relevant to this include (Sloan, 2004) 'stimuli for what is discussed during clinical supervision' and 'the routine'. 'The supervisor's approach' (Sloan, 2004) across all three teams implied control and direction of supervisees rather than promoting discovery and independence. There were many examples of supervisees taking issues to the clinical supervisor for approval. The emphasis placed on 'safety' appeared to thwart any opportunity of facilitating the supervisee's discovery and, instead, supervisors routinely provided answers.

Clinical supervision as a therapeutic endeavour

Opposing views have been presented in the psychotherapy literature concerning the therapeutic intentions of CS. Following many years of constructive debate, it is now generally understood as a means of developing practitioners' therapeutic integrity (Doehrmann, 1976; Loganbill et al., 1982; Bernard and Goodyear, 1998; Kilminster and Jolly, 2000). According to Watkins (1995), CS is a means of assisting a novice therapist to develop into an expert therapist rather than an expert client. If a trainee therapist requires therapy, they should be directed to this, but someone other than the clinical supervisor should provide it (Watkins, 1995). Supervision is not a replication of therapy. On the other hand, Davy (2002) highlights the considerable emphasis in the nursing literature on supervision as a personal support or stress-management mechanism for nurses. Several of the studies conducted previously, reviewed in Chapter 2, confirm this point.

Data from the present study are consistent with Davy's observations. The following quotes illuminate that CS was endorsed as a stress-relieving resource.

> Talking about stress, talking about difficulties within the team that I know David has no axe to grind on. So it's safe from that point of view. And I think I specifically used that when I came down here because I found it difficult to be honest . . . So I suppose initially I used David to offload a lot of that grief, which is possibly unfair to him, but he was the only person that I could do that with . . . professionally.
> (Case Site Two, 2nd interview with Nicola, supervisee and supervisor, 14/09/00 p. 4)

I think we benefit greatly from that wee bit of time out. Hopefully, the team benefits from a happier, less stressed . . . workforce . . . and obviously developing knowledge and whatever. Obviously, you do your job much better if you're feeling less stressed and had the opportunity to offload some stuff.
(Case Site Two, interview with Sarah, supervisor, 11/03/99 p. 19)

I try to get them just to explore their feelings. I think I use some of my counselling stuff just to get them to ventilate a wee bit – just to make them sure it's not threatening, it's not seen as a failing to have emotional feelings or stressed feelings about things. I just ask them how they feel about things and what brings these feelings on . . . I try to encourage them to talk about their feelings about the situation.
(Case Site Three, interview with Michael, clinical supervisor and team leader, 24/02/99 pp. 7–8)

The perception that supervision provided some level of therapeutic exchange was predominantly a feature of CS in Case Site One and Two. Managers and clinical supervisors, as highlighted by the following excerpts, appeared to sanction a therapeutic focus during supervision as a legitimate use of CS.

Maybe they have experienced . . . something that brought up . . . something for them, which . . . did happen . . . like: 'that was the way my father spoke to me', 'that is the way my husband speaks to me', and maybe a client has commented, 'I didn't like the way my father spoke to me', 'I didn't like the way my husband spoke to me', and that brought up again those feelings for them . . . What we look at is how they dealt with that and what feelings it brought up for them . . . I try to . . . question them more on the feelings that are around for themselves.
(Case Site One, interview with Megan, clinical supervisor, 11/03/99 p. 10)

The business that we do is highly emotive and we're trained to do it, but people can get emotional baggage; so I feel that it has a therapeutic . . . side as well that people can unload in that time their emotional baggage and receive that from their colleagues. So it's got a therapeutic value for the person: it's an offloading; it's therapy for them.
(Case Site Two, interview with Ross, team leader, 10/02/99 p. 8)

I think you know the type of job we are in. It is very easy for us to get engrossed in patients' problems and ignore our own. So in a way it's almost like the patient–nurse scenario.
(Interview with Jack, patient services manager, 04/02/99 p. 11)

The investigations conducted by Butterworth et al. (1997), Dunn (1998), Nicklin (1997b) and Teasdale et al. (1998) fail to provide evidence in support of focusing on nurses' welfare during CS. Fothergill et al. (2000) challenge further the idea of CS as a stress-reducing resource. This study, the largest survey to date of CMHNs' levels of stress, coping and burnout, identifies coping strategies used by nurses. These included diverting one's attention away from work, social support and a positive attitude towards one's role at work (Fothergill *et al.*, 2000). The nurses who participated in this study made no mention of the potential value of CS as a strategy to help them to cope with stress. More recently, Wright (2003) supports the use of expert counselling for nurses experiencing burnout. Like Fothergill *et al.* (2000), Wright (2003) makes no reference to CS or its value in this area.

Yegdich (1998, 1999b) challenges the assumption that CS can enhance both professional development and the emotional welfare of nurses. By combining the two processes of personal and professional growth into one, Yegdich (1999b) argues that a poor representation of both therapy and supervision is yielded. According to this psychotherapist, 'talking about patients and one's therapeutic work, in preference to oneself and one's personal issues, is the cornerstone of supervision' (Yegdich, 1999b, p. 1272).

According to Jones (1996), there are concerns regarding CS as a result of it being misunderstood as a form of enforced counselling or personal therapy. Wilkin *et al.* (1997) suggest that the perception of CS as a form of personal therapy may be one of the reasons for resistance to supervision. While this issue, up until now, has not been reported from any of the research conducted in nursing, it has emerged in recent research on supervision in counselling. Supervisees whose boundary between counselling and supervision was breached reported that this had been a disturbing and distressing experience (Kaberry, 2000). Moreover, those supervisees who had been subjected to personal counselling during their supervision had felt abused by the experience.

Some of the supervisees in the present study did not welcome CS having some level of therapeutic purpose. In particular, the supervisees in Case Site One commented on their negative experiences of Megan's attempts at merging supervision with therapy. Megan's own notions of supervision included an assumption that those for whom she provided supervision would accept that it had a therapeutic slant. According to all the supervisees in this team, this had never been discussed with them. Consequently, Megan's intention of CS having some level of therapeutic purpose to her supervisees was apparently exercised without collaboration or negotiation. Supervisees were uncomfortable with Megan's intrusive inquiry.

> I think there is a characteristic of Megan that is very nosy. I'm sure there is no harm meant from her, but it doesn't feel very nice. I want to say, 'I don't want to talk about that. That's not what I'm here for.'
> (Case Site One, 2nd interview with Lesley, supervisee, 29/03/01 p. 2)

> (*long, long pause*) I was thinking of one session, I think there is also a bit, it's like gossipy, it's like prying, it's like, there was something to do with these G-grade posts coming up . . . and she had asked me if I had thought of applying and I had said no, I had not thought about it, and (CPN colleague) had been in the building just prior to our meeting and he had been checking me out as well and I had felt sort of uneasy about that and so during supervision I had said, 'Oh, that's funny

(CPN colleague) had been asking me that.' Before I knew it, it was weedled out of me what I was thinking about it. It was like I suddenly found myself saying something I did not want to say, but it wasn't relevant.
(Case Site One, interview with Rachel, supervisee, 03/02/99 p. 10)

To be honest, it wasn't helpful, and I came out thinking I had let Megan know what was going on, but I'd felt as if I was being questioned. There was a nosy aspect to it. I thought, 'Well, I won't do that again.' You know, not going into great detail about stuff.
(Case Site One, interview with Georgie, supervisee, 28/03/01 p. 9)

Findings from the present study highlighting that CS had therapeutic connotations would appear to illuminate how current conceptual ambiguities pervade clinical practice. Ultimately, coinciding with other diversions, this distracted those engaging in supervision from its other tasks. In nursing, policy makers in the UK expected that CS would contribute towards improvements in patient care (DoH, 1993; UKCC, 1996). In mental health nursing, CS is expected to enhance and develop competence in nurses' therapeutic contact with patients (Termini and Hauser, 1973; Benfer, 1979; CPNA, 1985; Critchley, 1987; Farkas-Cameron, 1995). The following section illustrates the extent to which client-related issues featured in supervision.

Client-related issues: absence of relating to the client

Findings from all three teams highlighted that clinical issues, and specifically client-related issues, were brought to supervision. Discussion of clients was of a brief nature, similar to that commonly known as the traditional ward handover. In the context of the ward handover, the information conveyed by the nurse reporting on patients is for the benefit of the recipients – those listening to the report in preparation for taking over the care of patients.

Some of the participants had some ideas as to the reasons for this occurring in CS. In the following excerpts, Scott and Gillian, supervisees from Case Site One, share their opinions.

The purpose . . . I think is partly to keep up with what is happening in (team base). To keep a finger on what's happening with everyone's caseloads, with individuals who are attending, with the groups, what people are involved in . . . There is this feeling around and it's maybe just to keep tabs on everything that's happening.
(Case Site One, interview with Scott, supervisee, 10/03/99 p. 12)

I was told at the beginning, you know, 'I've been doing supervision for four years and this is how I do it; we go over your caseload and then we have an opportunity to talk about anything else that you feel is pertinent.'
(Case Site One, interview with Gillian, supervisee, 23/03/01 p. 9)

These opinions are supported by data that emerged from CS session documents and audio-recordings of supervision.

> Format somewhat predetermined. Went through client caseload briefly.
> (Case Site One, clinical supervision session record, Scott, supervisee, 01/04/99)

Gillian	Right, well (client A), you know that he's changed his days and we're trying to get him along on other days as well?
Megan	Yes.
Gillian	So you know all about him. (Client T) will be reviewed today. I discharged that chap there. I'll need to score that off. This lady is doing really well. She comes to the women's group.
Megan	She's doing extremely well, isn't she?
Gillian	Oh, she's doing great. These are all outreach people so they will be starting when the outreach starts. They need the dates for that.
Megan	(Client B) comes into anxiety management?
Gillian	Yes. These two (*pointing to client list*) are outreach. I've never had the chance to update this. I've got patients that aren't even on that. She's in the anxiety group. She's my main concern because of her physical health really but we discussed that today. (Client A) as you know is getting quite dependent and is giving different messages to different people. (Occupational therapist colleague) did a home assessment and he giggled all the way through it. He's been asking (CPN colleague) if he could come here a few extra days and I'm just really trying not to let him do that. He's good for the Christmas concert and we appreciate his keyboard playing and one thing and another but I think he could get his feet under the table very quickly so we need to watch that and tell him when his time is up. I'm going to try and get him to engage in the outreach at (community resource).

(Case Site One, audio-recording with Megan and Gillian, 16/10/00 pp. 1–3)

The following example illustrates how Stephanie reported back on several clients within a short period of time.

Stephanie	(*laughing*) (Client AC) . . . is one of (colleagues) I saw the other day. She's just needing a wee bit of support through the next couple of weeks. (Client AD) . . . is a chap with symptoms of depression and he's just been started on an antidepressant. I've made an outpatient appointment for him. He needs a lot of reassurance. I'm looking at his notes just now and he's got a lot of biological symptoms of depression and it's not just the way he is thinking. So he's got an outpatient appointment. (*medium pause*) That's that guy we were talking about today. (Client F) (is) a woman who was in (hospital ward) because there were no beds. It wasn't that she qualified for a bed in (hospital ward). She was referred back to the home option team form (hospital ward), which shouldn't be done.

(Case Site Two, audio-recording with David and Stephanie, 15/01/01 pp. 4–5)

On a minority of occasions, the supervisee expanded their report. Nonetheless, the content of these reports generally centred around the assessment of a client's mental health, liaising with colleagues, medication issues and issues relating to clients' discharge. On the other hand, discussion on the nurse–client relationship was absent, as was the therapeutic intentions of nurses' contact with clients.

While focusing on CS, the present study uncovered the limited extent to which these mental health nurses engaged in discussions concerning therapeutic interventions. There is potential therapeutic gain from nurses engaging with patients for the purposes of assessment, liaising with colleagues and discharge; nonetheless, the lack of any evidence of discussion on the therapeutic nurse–patient relationship or intentional therapeutic interventions must be acknowledged. Findings relevant to this theme reflect earlier work. Studies of psychiatric nursing practice during the past 30 years have consistently identified the fact that nurses tend not to demonstrate or acknowledge their contribution towards therapeutic interventions (Altschul, 1972; Cormack, 1976; Cormack, 1983; Gijbels, 1995; Bray, 1999). This might imply, as suggested by Sullivan (1998) and Laurance (2003), that there was no appreciation of the concept of nurse–patient interactions in the clinical practice of mental health nursing. Alternatively, perhaps supervisees felt unable to disclose aspects of their involvement with patients because of how supervision was provided in these teams. They may have felt under pressure to show that they were managing their caseloads, which emerged as a priority for clinical supervisors, and therefore avoided sharing the intricacies of their relationships with patients.

The broad scope of clinical supervision

There appears to be some endorsement in the nursing literature of the notion that there are no boundaries as to what can be discussed during CS. McEvoy (1993) reports that personal needs, worries or problems at work could be discussed in CS. Fowler (1996c) describes how supervision could be used for the catharsis of distress resulting from failing to get a promotion. Reports of 'life events' being discussed during CS have been published (Rafferty and Coleman, 1996). Supervisee reflections have highlighted that staff relations and tensions amongst professional colleagues were discussed during supervision (Hadfield and Booton, 2003). It is therefore perhaps no surprise that the majority of participants across the three teams in the present study understood CS as an opportunity to discuss 'Affairs, Sexual Dysfunctions and Anything Else' and 'Anything and Everything' (Sloan, 2004).

The following examples, from Case Site Two, illustrate how CS provided participants with an opportunity to discuss 'Affairs, Sexual Dysfunctions and Anything Else'.

My experience of it here has been that it's been anything that I've wanted it to be.
(Case Site Two, interview with Callum, supervisee, 05/04/99 p. 12)

If there's anything worrying him, if there's anything, you know, any issues that he is not happy about or wants to discuss . . .
(Case Site Two, interview with Sarah, supervisor, 11/03/99 p. 1)

I know that it's an opportunity to bring up anything and David always asks me if there is anything outwith my caseload that I want to discuss but there never has been, but I know there is an opportunity to bring things up if I wanted to.
(Case Site Two, interview with Stephanie, supervisee, 23/03/01 p. 1)

. . . and then I want to open it out to her and let her bring anything that she has.
(Case Site Two, interview with David, supervisor and supervisee,
01/03/99 p. 5)

The more you get . . . to know people, supervision is a formal aspect but . . . we all have personal problems and we all try to get in there and put a big professional face on it. If you can get a good therapeutic relationship with someone and they feel trusted and valued with you, I have dealt with and I know that supervisors have dealt with some really emotive things in people's lives whereas, if it was just a formal structure, you know, too clinical, you know that would be overlooked; they wouldn't even share that with you; so, if it's working really well and you . . . feel confident and (*brief pause*) feel that they can, they will share some things that are happening . . . So, if it's working really well, I think we can practise what we preach a lot of the time if it's working really well because that's hard to say, you know, if your marriage is breaking up or you're impotent or whatever, getting any-thing like that, you know, just, financial debt or you're having an affair . . . things like that . . . if they feel that it won't go any further and things like that, that it can, you know, come into their personal life and shouldn't be naive, you know, we all have areas in our life that we can all get (*quietly spoken*) depressed, anxious and all of the problems and relationship problems.
(Case Site Two, interview with Ross, team leader, 10/02/99 p. 27)

I think a danger is that you narrowly only talk about their caseload. It is making sure that they realise that they can talk about absolutely anything. They can talk about problems at home if need be.
(Interview with Jack, patient services manager, 04/02/99 p. 6)

CS may have been seen as an opportunity to discuss supervisees' personal experiences because of a lack of other avenues. Managerial supervision and staff welfare, support and education are, as clarified earlier, the essential foun-dations upon which CS can flourish (Yegdich, 1999b). The majority of partic-ipants commented that there was an absence of opportunities outwith of CS to discuss line-management issues. The work of Cpns is often conducted in isolation, and these nurses can work from day to day with little contact with colleagues. There is a need to create opportunities that demonstrate staff welfare and support but which are distinguishable from the purposes of CS.

The time afforded to the discussion of those items resulting from the broad scope of CS limited the time available to discuss client-related issues. In the present study, supervisory discussions were filled with 'Anything and Everything' (Sloan, 2004) thus limiting the time available for any focused exploration of clinical practice. Yet, reflecting on one's clinical work demands, amongst other things, time (Johns, 1997; Todd and Freshwater, 1999; Rolfe *et al.*, 2001).

OBJECTIVE 2

To explore and describe supervisees' experiences of individual CS.

None of the supervisees reported having had the opportunity to express their views on the provision of CS, and none recalled being asked for feedback on their supervisory experiences. It is possible that there was some degree of complacency concerning CS; it happened and so there was no need to delve deeper. Consequently, the opportunity they were afforded during the research may have contributed to the rich textures within the data. The majority of participants had experienced a particular format for the delivery of supervision. In all three teams 'the routine' (Sloan, 2004) indicated long-standing rituals in its provision.

The routine: hierarchy

The use of hierarchy in the context of CS in each of the three teams had been defended for many years. Rebecca (SM) had introduced CS in this way around 1985 and her supervisees from that period, now TLs in CMHTs, maintained its hierarchical provision. However, human resources for community services had increased substantially, and the teams included nurses on grades ranging from H-grade to B-grade. Accordingly, as illustrated by the following excerpts, the TLs (H grade) would line manage the CNs (G grade); the CNs would line manage the SNs (E grade), and the SNs would line manage the nursing assistants (B grade).

I think Rebecca made the initial set up, which would be (during) early nineties, probably earlier than that, who set up supervision and she supervised us initially as G grades on a monthly basis. Probably, that is how it happened. We would then do the same. Rebecca was the patient services manager or nursing officer, I can't remember what the title was then – clinical nurse manager. That is what she was. And I think we took a lead from that because that was the first time we had experienced supervision, and then we just followed on with monthly (frequency of CS).
(Interview with Jack, patient services manager, 04/02/99 pp. 1–2)

Ross will supervise the charge nurses. He is the team leader. The charge nurses will supervise the staff nurses. We have a nursing assistant. One of the staff nurses will supervise her, you know; it's laid down . . . in that structure. It's not through choice or anything, you know. I supervise Nicola because she is my staff nurse.
(Case Site Two, interview with David, clinical supervisor, 01/03/99 p. 5)

So it was a hierarchical clinical supervision method: it was the Gs supervising the Es, supervising the Bs.
(Interview with Emma, patient services manager, 18/03/99 p. 2)

CS was regarded as part of line-management responsibilities. Consequently, in all three teams there was a powerful managerial influence over participants' engagement in CS.

Yet, UKCC (1996) stresses that CS should not be delivered by hierarchy. Furthermore, CS should not be confused with a form of managerial control that incorporated managerial responsibility and supervision. Similar guidelines were included in the Division's document for CS (Appendix One). It would appear that these guidelines could not penetrate the central characteristics and ritualised format of 'the routine' (Sloan, 2004).

Concerns have been expressed as a consequence of CS being misunderstood (Burrow, 1995; Cotton, 2001; Gilbert, 2001). CS is frequently resisted because of the perception that it is something that is provided by a supervisor who has a hierarchical and managerial function over the supervisee (Wilkin *et al.*, 1997; Duarri and Kendrick, 1999; Gilbert, 2001). When this occurs, there is a structural power differential and often an appraisal function that accompanies the role of clinical supervisor. While 'dual role incompatibility' was prominent in Case Site One (Sloan, 2004), the tensions created as a result of CS being provided by a line manager also resonated throughout the findings peculiar to Case Site Two and Three. It became apparent that both clinical supervisors and supervisees contributed to 'dual role incompatibility'.

In the following excerpt, Heather describes how her clinical supervisor/line manager leads the process of CS.

I sort of follow Michael's lead at the moment; he kind of sets the objectives and agenda.
(Case Site Three, interview with Heather, supervisee, 24/02/99 p. 2)

In the following example, in explaining what she was looking for from Megan on this particular occasion, Lesley describes how she, as the supervisee, could contribute to 'dual role incompatibility'.

I think support for me because I think I was feeling quite isolated. Myself and (colleague) had been there the longest and (colleague) had been there two years. I don't know why, but I just felt quite alone and needed a wee bit of support, encouragement and reassurance as well that she had it in hand and she knew what was going to happen. I don't feel she did have that in hand, and it felt all over the place. It felt we were just out on a limb somewhere and nobody was really containing it because I don't think she was in control of it. I don't think she has much control in (team base) in respect of who comes and who goes. I think there are other things that influence that. So I was looking for a wee bit of reassurance that things were going to be OK and they were going to be OK because, 'this is what we are going to do and this is what we can do and what would you like to happen!' (Case Site One, 2nd interview with Lesley, supervisee, 29//03/01 p. 8)

The following example from an audio-recording, one from a considerable quantity which was gathered from Megan's provision of supervision to all supervisees, illustrates the combined influence the supervisee and supervisor had on this predicament. Gillian checked out the continued support for a new group from her CN. This is highlighted by the italicised sections of the text. Megan, as CN, gave her support; these sections are also in italics.

Gillian   *And are you still on*; it will be sorted out hopefully tomorrow one way or another but I do feel that the amount of referrals are coming from (addictions unit) for this discharge group, it's a bug bear of mine just now but the referrals have certainly dwindled from . . .
Megan   *I'll support you.*
Gillian   I think really there is a definite need for something like a wee group like that but as you know it's been on hold until we have this meeting with the community mental health teams and get them involved.
Megan   I mean *I'll support you on that, Gillian*, in giving out PR to these folk. (Case Site One, Megan and Gillian, audio-recording, 11/04/00 p. 21)

In Case Site Two, having acknowledged these tensions, a small number of participants made attempts at 'going against the routine' (Sloan, 2004). In the following excerpt, Sarah discloses how she arranged alternative opportunities for CS, engaging in peer supervision with a colleague working in another community mental health team.

But . . . at one time I had sought out a supervisor from the other team because I felt the need for supervision and I wasn't getting it where I was so I had sought out another G grade from another team, which was extremely useful, and it kind of helped for a period of time, and this need sort of stopped . . . I'd say the need is probably back again but, or has been back again, but maybe (the) opportunity hasn't been there . . . I felt I gained a lot more. I felt I learned, I really learned, a lot on clinical issues . . . It wasn't known about (*quietly spoken, giggling*) . . . It was known about from their side but not from this side. (Case Site Two, interview with Sarah, clinical supervisor, 11/03/99 p. 23)

Supervisees in this study were told who would be their clinical supervisor despite the Division's document on CS encouraging supervisees to have some degree of choice. There is considerable support for supervisees having some choice of their clinical supervisor (UKCC, 1996; Kipping, 1998; May, 2003; Cerinus, 2003; Edwards *et al.*, 2005). Mullarkey *et al.* (2001) go as far as to suggest that giving supervisees the freedom to choose their supervisor should be a key principle for CS. They argue that this choice should be based on their own identified needs and also the skills and experience of the supervisor.

However, facilitating alternative arrangements for CS instead of a hierarchical provision is not without complications. A possible option is the creation of a database of supervisors (Jones, 2001a). Supervisors could be included on the database providing they met certain criteria, for example some level of training in supervision and previous supervisory experience. Information maintained about supervisors could include their availability, professional background, additional training, supervisory training and experience and areas of particular interest. The supervisee and supervisor would have an opportunity to meet and determine if they could work together prior to making a formalised agreement (Sloan, 2005).

The frequency and duration of sessions

The influence of hierarchy was not the only feature that remained from the early stages of the introduction of CS. Rebecca provided supervision to her G grades on a monthly basis usually lasting an hour. An aspect of 'the routine' for all of the teams in the current study related to the frequency and duration of supervision. There appeared to be little variation amongst supervision pairs regarding the frequency and duration of individual sessions.

In Case Site One and Two, supervision was intended to be provided on a monthly basis and last for an hour.

Well, usually at the end of each supervision session we arrange it for a month, sort of four-weekly down the line. So we just do that at the end of each session. It's monthly, yes. I think we set aside an hour.
(Case Site One, interview with Lesley, supervisee, 17/02/99 p. 1)

I put an hour by for a session of supervision . . . Well, just now it's monthly.
(Case Site One, interview with Megan, supervisor, 11/03/99 pp. 1–2)

The way it's been organised . . . has been, I've had supervision about once every four weeks.
(Case Site Two, interview with Callum, supervisee, 05/04/99 p. 1)

We meet monthly. We aim at an hour and it sometimes goes over that; it's no more than an hour and a half.
(Case Site Two, interview with Sarah, supervisor, 11/03/99 pp. 1–2)

These stipulations correspond, to some extent, with the results of the validation study of the Manchester Clinical Supervision Scale (Winstanley and White,

2003), which recommend that supervision should be provided on a monthly basis. Nevertheless, they do not correspond with the recommendation that, for community-based staff, CS sessions should extend beyond an hour (Winstanley and White, 2003). In Case Site Three, CS was provided on a two-monthly basis and usually lasted 45 minutes, which is also not consistent with these recommendations. More importantly, perhaps the frequency and duration of sessions should be negotiated between the clinical supervisor and supervisee according to individual need. The extent of the supervisee's experience, complexity of clinical issues, nature of the work and other commitments should have some bearing on these arrangements. In a recent study aimed at identifying the factors that may influence the effectiveness of CS for community mental health nurses in Wales, in keeping with the recommendations suggested by Winstanley and White (2003), CS was more positively evaluated where sessions lasted for over an hour and took place on at least a once-monthly basis (Edwards *et al.*, 2005).

The supervisor's agenda

In each of the teams, the supervisor's agenda had a significant influence over discussions. The clinical supervisor's agenda took precedence. In Case Site One, 'keeping the supervisor up to date using the client list' and 'staff relationship issues and personal issues' (Sloan, 2004) were dominant items on Megan's agenda.

Data from audio-recordings of CS illuminate Megan's adherence to her agenda and quintessence of 'keeping the supervisor up-to-date using the client list'. The examples presented are typical of the considerable portion emerging from this site.

Lesley   Client wise there's nothing really (*brief pause*). (Client D) is in the assertive skills and is fine. (Client L) didn't come yesterday but she's coming today to get her bloods checked for her Lithium levels.
Megan   What was wrong with her, Lesley?
Lesley   Nothing, she'd been working. She'd to do a night shift and then had to do extra hours in the morning. (Client G) will be in today. (Client E) is pretty down but . . . if she comes in. (Client J) is in the assertive-skills group, and she is doing really well. (Client S), well, you heard about (client S) yesterday. He's a wee darling. I don't know much else; I don't really see him regularly at all to be honest. It's (colleague) that sees him regularly. (Client A) he's in the art group and he's fine. (Client Y) should be in today at some point. That chap (client D) I took on didn't come yesterday.
(Case Site One, audio-recording with Megan and Lesley, 02/02/01 pp. 2–4)

Holly   On the list of clients, these are the ones I've discharged . . . This lady's in hospital but I was thinking about discharging her but when she's a bit better she'll start attending from hospital probably as preparation for discharge, like she did the last time.

Megan   I would agree with you there, Holly, because she's actually been out in the past now. I checked that out yesterday.
Holly   Yeah.
Megan   And she's a good bit better from what she was and that's something the ward was sort of thinking that she would maybe just tap back into (team base) again.
Holly   Yeah.
Megan   I said to them the space was open, which we discussed anyway.
Holly   Yeah.
Megan   So the space was open.
Holly   The third lady . . . didn't keep the appointment and I contacted her, but she's doing well, and I made sure with Gillian that she really was doing well. So we're just going to leave it until the end. She's really fine and (session interrupted). It's proved really beneficial and she's got absolutely no problems; so we're just leaving that. This gentleman was waiting to go to the next anxiety management. Now this gentleman I finished up actually discharging last week because he was supposed to start the structured group and he didn't. He identified that he had got physical abuse going on when he was a child and we explored all kinds of avenues to get assistance with that.
Megan   Yes?
Holly   (*sighing*) This chap's still in the structured group. He'd wanted the anxiety management but he's declined that now and his attendance for the structured group is less and less; so I think once that's finished we won't be going much further than that. Number seven, he is in the structured group and he's beginning to address, he kept talking about this issue when he was in the Marines and he actually offloaded it on Tuesday and you could see him physically better because he'd actually managed to discuss it . . . Yeah, and we're both taking the same tack with him that, 'OK your physical health is a big issue', you can't deny this because he's been in so much pain but that's not going to change so you know, 'how do we make the best of your health and how can we move forward with your health?', in that way, but we also need to sort of address these issues from the past; so we've been on the same wavelength and it's working. The next three people, these are long-term patients that I got from Lesley. I met this gentleman just to sort of let him know who his keyworker is at the moment. He's got no real problems at the moment, but we've left it that if he wants any help he'll call me.

(Case Site One, audio-recording with Megan and Holly, 20/04/00 pp. 1–4)

Some writers assert the opportunity to focus on clinical issues and develop skills as a benefit to the supervisee, the recipient of CS (Dudley and Butterworth, 1994; Styles and Gibson, 1999; Veeramah, 2002). It is difficult to appreciate how the supervisee benefited from engaging in such a superficial exchange regardless of the focus being on clients. Furthermore, any benefit for the clinical supervisor was equally limited.

The other essential item on Megan's agenda related to prompting supervisees to feedback on 'staff relationship issues and personal issues' (Sloan, 2004). Supervisees could recount many examples of such discussions.

If I'm honest with you, it tends to become very general with supervision, you know, I go off and talk about something completely different. Megan maybe asks about my family or this, that and the next thing, you know, and I've encouraged that, I must admit.
(Case Site One, interview with Jordan, supervisee, 25/03/99 p. 5)

It has tended to be about personality clashes and when I've felt I've been put under pressure. We've had a lot of problems in relation to outreach. There was an understanding by Gillian and myself that we were employed for outreach because that's what the job description and the job advert said and so we thought that's what we had been employed for. The rest of the team had thought we were employed to come to (team base) and be just two of the staff doing outreach. They had an expectation that it would rotate, and everybody who wanted a turn at outreach would get that, and Gillian and myself were . . . a little surprised . . . putting it mildly. Now that was discussed at length outwith supervision as well as during supervision.
(Case Site One, interview with Holly, supervisee, 26/03/01 pp. 8–9)

'Caseload numbers' and 'professional development' (Sloan, 2004) were agenda items in Case Site Two, which David referred to frequently. David explains:

I like to think that I leave the agenda to Nicola, but these are things that I want to know, you know. I want to know what her caseload is; I want to know what her case mix is; I want to know how she is getting on with the GPs.
(Case Site Two, interview with David, supervisor and supervisee, 01/03/99 p. 5)

In the following example, David's agenda is illustrated in CS with Stephanie.

Stephanie	I'll just go through my caseload. I can't think of any particular problems with anybody; so I'll just go through it to remind myself.
David	What's your caseload numbers just now?
Stephanie	It's about 35 I think.
David	35, is that including the groups?
Stephanie	Yes.
David	How many have you got in your groups?
Stephanie	About a dozen.

(Case Site Two, audio-recording with David and Stephanie, 24/03/00 p. 1)

Finally, in Case Site Three 'the clinical supervision support form' (Sloan, 2004) was used by Daniel to influence issues discussed during CS.

Same procedure as the last time on the form here.
(Case Site Three, audio-recording with Daniel and Claire, 29/08/00 p. 1)

The 'supervision support form' had the headings 'caseload/mix', 'case presentations', 'relations with staff', 'job satisfaction/reflection of work', 'personal

You know if I had a problem with a client I would take it to the Kardex; I wouldn't take it to Megan.
(Case Site One, interview with Gillian, supervisee, 23/03/01 p. 10)

Whereas I have no worries about what I would take to my external supervision, where there is nothing I wouldn't take to it, that feels so safe . . . It is just, the first thing is the safety.
(Case Site One, interview with Rachel, supervisee, 03/02/99 pp. 11–12)

While there have been reports of the barriers to implementing CS, there is less written about the negative experiences of nurses during CS in the nursing literature. Notable exceptions include the work on mental health nurses by Scanlon and Weir (1997), Kipping (1998) and Duncan-Grant (2000a) and a study of a general nursing setting reported by O'Riordan (2002). According to Scanlon and Weir (1997) and Kipping (1998), the CS experienced by the majority of mental health nurses in these studies was regarded as unhelpful. But it is O'Riordan (2002) who identifies that staff withdrew from CS as a result of the clinical supervisor being an insider to the unit and that it was hierarchical, higher grades supervising lower grades. The behaviours described by supervisees in Case Site One are similar to those described in a study of supervision of clinical psychologists. Greer (2002) describes how clinical psychologists turned to other peers when experiencing inadequate supervision.

Conversely, supervisees working in Case Site Two and Three spoke favourably of their CS experiences. They valued having the opportunity to engage in supervision. They all spoke highly of each of their clinical supervisors. These supervisees did not express the view that their supervision had been compromised because it had been provided by their line manager. Despite this, tensions relating to the provision of CS, albeit to a lesser extent than supervisees in Case Site One, were raised in Case Site Two and Three. The categories 'going against the routine' (Sloan, 2004) in Case Site Two and 'an evolving process' (Sloan, 2004) in Case Site Three illuminated how team members, in acknowledging their negative experiences with 'the routine', challenged the provision of CS (Sloan, 2004).

The following example illustrates a TL's ideas about giving supervisees some choice in their clinical supervisor and that this person did not necessarily have to be their line manager.

I think it's being looked at just now as it could be improved upon; someone could actually select another staff nurse.
(Case Site Three, interview with Liam, team leader, 25/03/99 p. 1)

Neither clinical supervisors nor supervisees in any of the teams were given the opportunity to provide feedback and review their experiences of CS. This would appear to be an important consideration, particularly when the experience is less than helpful. Nonetheless, the opportunity to review supervision when it appears to be working well is also necessary since tensions can exist during the delivery of what seems to be helpful supervision.

Acknowledging participants' need to review their experiences of engaging in CS has been emphasised in some of the supervision contract templates published in the supervision literature. In particular, Howard's (1997) supervisory agreement encourages the supervisor and supervisee to frequently evaluate their experiences of CS (Sloan, 2005).

OBJECTIVE 3

To describe how the organisational provision of CS influences the supervisory process.

It has been argued that the context in which CS exists affects its nature and processes (Bond and Holland, 1998). As highlighted in Chapter 2, few nurse researchers have addressed this aspect in previous investigations. In the current study, three categories – (Sloan, 2004) 'the stimuli for what is discussed during clinical supervision', 'preparation for clinical supervision' and 'the routine' – emerged that illuminate the organisational provision for CS and its influence on the supervisory process. With 'the routine' having been described earlier, the two remaining categories will be clarified.

The stimuli for what is discussed during clinical supervision

Recurring themes (Sloan, 2004) for the category 'the stimuli for what is discussed during clinical supervision' across all teams included 'problems' and 'doing the right thing'. CS was regarded as an opportunity to deal with any problems that a supervisee might have experienced. Managers and clinical supervisors thought that dealing with 'problems' would ensure supervisees were 'doing the right thing'. While there is general agreement that supervision in nursing provides an opportunity to discuss problems (Butterworth et al., 1998a; Adcock, 1999; Cheater and Hale, 2001), if given too much of a priority, this could limit the potential benefit of CS.

The focus on problems appeared to have a strong influence from management sources, for example Jack (PSM) and Rebecca (SM).

> So I think patients would only be discussed if they were seen as a problem.
> (Interview with Jack, patient services manager, 04/02/99 p. 1)

> I would encourage individuals to come to me with areas of difficulty first of all, you know, where they were struggling.
> (Interview with Rebecca, senior manager, 10/05/99 p. 5)

Likewise, supervisees acknowledged that CS was somewhere to take their problems.

If I was having a problem with a client in any way – attendance or if they were bringing problems I didn't know how to deal with.
(Case Site One, interview with Holly, supervisee, 26/03/01 p. 8)

An area to sort of troubleshoot any problems I suppose.
(Case Site Two, interview with Nicola, supervisee and supervisor, 11/02/99 p. 3)

I've been settling in. We've had teething problems and it's . . . a good opportunity to look at how we can make sure things run smoothly.
(Case Site Three, interview with Louise, supervisee, 03/03/99 and 07/04/99 p. 2)

For some authors, CS was intended to create an opportunity for practitioners to reflect on their delivery of therapeutic approaches and not necessarily focus on good or bad practice (Loganbill *et al.*, 1982; Minot and Adamski, 1989; Rankin, 1989; Bernard and Goodyear, 1998; Yegdich, 1999b). With so much emphasis being placed on identifying and resolving problems in each of the teams in the current study, there appeared to be only a limited opportunity for nurses to reflect on their relationships with patients or acknowledge, celebrate and learn from examples of good practice. Furthermore, in nursing, CS is also thought to provide a forum where good practices can be confirmed and praised (Faugier and Butterworth, 1994; Palsson *et al.*, 1994; Begat *et al.*, 1997; Jones, 1997; Arvidsson *et al.*, 2000; Hadfield, 2000), something that was observed infrequently in the present study.

'Doing the right thing' (Sloan, 2004) appeared to have some connection with ensuring safe practice. The emphasis placed on safety, however, appeared to reduce the opportunities for exploration and reflection of clinical practice. There were limited opportunities for facilitating supervisees' reflections on 'good enough' practices, yet widespread endorsement of clinical supervisors ensuring that supervisees were 'doing the right thing'. The following excerpts illustrate the emphasis given to 'doing the right thing' by supervisees and a clinical supervisor.

That staff are doing the right things with clients.
(Case Site One, interview with Megan, clinical supervisor, 11/03/99 p. 5)

So I really go to my supervision looking to see if I'm on the right track and if there's anything I can do, you know, to change it or make it better.
(Case Site Three, interview with Iona, supervisee, 07/04/99 p. 2)

I think I feel, I don't know. (*brief pause*) I think I feel I need to know myself that I am doing the right thing or going about something in the right way.
(Case Site One, interview with Hannah, supervisee, 05/03/99 p. 16)

It was the psychoanalyst Donald Winnicott who introduced the concept of the 'good enough mother' (Hawkins and Shohet, 2000). The concept makes reference to the mother who, when her child rejects her caring, does not over-react or sink under feelings of inadequacy but can perceive this event as her child expressing its temporary inability to cope (Winnicott, 1965). In these cir-cumstances, Winnicott (1965) suggest that it is difficult for any mother to be 'good enough' unless she herself is supported. This concept provides a useful analogy for CS where the 'good enough' nurse can survive the tensions within her relationships with patients through the supervisory relationship. Yet, in these teams, it would appear that expectations of supervisees appeared to exceed being 'good enough'.

The Allitt Inquiry (Clothier et al., 1994) concluded that the lack of man-agerial supervision in the children's wards at Grantham and Kesteven General Hospitals contributed to the deaths and injuries caused by a nurse. However, DoH (1993) and UKCC (1996) propose CS as a strategy to ensure consumer protection. Following on from this, it is suggested that CS can function as a risk-management tool (Tingle, 1995; Walker and Clark, 1999; Herron, 2000). It is therefore perhaps understandable that CS represented a means of ensuring nurses were 'doing the right thing' and practising safely.

Preparation for clinical supervision

Previous experiences of receiving clinical supervision

In all three teams, participants had limited preparation for their engagement in CS. The majority of participants relied on their own previous experiences of receiving supervision to guide their own delivery. Thus, supervisees in the present study received supervision from their managers, who in turn had received supervision from their managers. The study site appeared to reflect Holyoake's (2000) observation that no formal qualifications or training are necessarily expected of clinical supervisors.

Driscoll (2000a) suggests that nurses have many skills that can be trans-ferred from the clinical setting to CS. Participants from Case Site Two and Three commented that the skills they used with patients were also used in supervision.

> To be honest, it was something I found very difficult to begin with. I was quite intimidated by it, especially when I kind of read things and everything, you know. I kind of tried to base it on some of the positive experiences I'd had of it and not do some of the negative things that I'd had as well as.
> (Case Site Two, interview with Sarah, supervisor, 11/03/99 p. 3)

> I have had a wide range of supervisory experiences both in hospital and in the community and I have had supervisory experiences that I would not wish on anyone else, but I've also had really good supervision sessions that I would like to think I could pass on to other people. But again this comes back to (*brief pause*); to be able to pass that on, you've really got to have had the experience of having

of this information generally related to supervisors sharing factual information concerning clients, their thoughts and opinions about clients and operational aspects relating to particular Trust procedures.

Lesley   I mean I did, on last Thursday, I did say to him, you know, I really kind of made him think about what he was getting from the sessions because I was a bit honest with him that I didn't know that I was able to give him much and because the last three appointments that he hasn't turned up for or he's phoned up heavily under the influence of alcohol and there's nothing that we can do and . . . I felt that this session we really needed to discuss that; so I think he was a bit taken aback and said, 'Oh, I'm shocked at that', you know and I explained, 'It's my opinion and I feel I've got to be honest with you.' By the end of it, he was saying he gets a lot from coming, even for a few days he's just dropped in for a coffee.

Megan   I've noticed him in. I think being honest with him has maybe achieved some change . . . There's nothing else you can do really.

(Case Site One, audio-recording with Megan and Lesley, 26/08/99 p. 7)

In the preceding example, there were opportunities for Megan to share theoretical and empirical information relating to establishing therapeutic alliances with clients, determining clients' motivation for engaging in a helping relationship or the contribution of motivational interviewing for people with alcohol-related difficulties. Alternatively, Megan could have utilised her own personal experiences of working with clients with similar issues as a means of sharing information with Lesley.

Many of the information-giving interactions appeared to relate to the clinical supervisors as managers, for example explaining what they would do as manager, sharing information regarding off-duty and annual leave or providing information about service developments. In the following example, Daniel informs Claire about his plans for new office premises.

Daniel   Oh yes, what I intend to do is actually to hold an office here.
Claire   Right.
Daniel   It might not be the one we're in.
Claire   Yeah.
Daniel   It might be next door. But the point you've got to look at there though, Claire, is that . . .
Claire   We don't need three bases with notes, do we?
Daniel   Now this is why I'm asking people to actually think about this. You know, you've maybe touched on them already. Are we going to end up with notes in three different places or in four different bases? No, not quite, but I think the main thing that I would be asking you to consider is the main base would, geographically, not be central.
Claire   That's right.
Daniel   And I think that's the problem. I think it's very good to have satellite bases, that is an office you can go and sit in and, say for example, in (local village)

it's great to have that office in there where (colleague) and (colleague) can geographically fit their visits in. But to actually have something like that as being your main base?

Claire   No.

Daniel   I think you could find it could cause great difficulties.

Claire   Yeah.

Daniel   And you're highlighting one there: where do we keep all the notes? Because effectively what we'd need to say is we generally need to keep the notes at our main base.

Claire   Yes.

Daniel   In (local village).

Claire   Yeah.

Daniel   Whereas the main base at the moment is (local village); it's geographically central when you're literally going through (local village).

(Case Site Three, audio-recording with Daniel and Claire, 27/10/00 p. 25)

The source of knowledge shared during CS in the present study was primarily personal, practical knowledge. All of the supervisors shared what they had done or gave their own opinion on particular situations. This type of knowledge does have an important contribution for a wide variety of nursing contexts (Burnard, 2002). Imparting other forms of knowledge was less evident. Furthermore, no reference was made by any of the participants to empirical literature, yet it has been suggested that there are important links to be established between CS and clinical governance (Lyle, 1998b; Redfern, 1998; Lipp and Osborne, 2000). Butterworth and Woods (1999) argue that both could work together to ensure safe and accountable practice.

The nursing literature is full of articles that describe a multitude of barriers to the dissemination of research in nursing and the principles of evidence-based practice. The reasons for this are complex and according to Hunt's (1987) influential paper include:

• nurses do not know about research findings;
• nurses do not understand the research process and findings;
• nurses do not believe research findings;
• nurses do not know how to apply research findings;
• nurses are not allowed to use research findings.

Consequently, it has been stressed that research findings are having little appreciable impact on nursing practice (McIntosh, 1995; McSherry, 1997; Nagy et al., 2001). It has been highlighted by McCloughen (2001) that the challenge of evidence-based nursing has frequently gone unheeded by mental health nurses. According to Ward et al. (2000), there is a lack of awareness of both qualitative and quantitative research methods and this results in an uncritical acceptance by mental health nurses of published material.

It seems plausible that those mental health nurses who take on the role of clinical supervisor may also have difficulties with introducing aspects relating to research into their CS discussions for reasons similar to those listed above. Before CS can make an appreciable contribution to the clinical-governance agenda, it is probable that practitioners will require assistance in overcoming these barriers. Otherwise, there will continue to be overconfidence in experiential knowledge (Thompson, 2003).

Agreeing with the supervisee

The approach of 'agreeing with the supervisee' (Sloan, 2004) appeared to be used frequently by supervisors to affirm and confirm something the supervisee had said or done. An earlier study investigating group supervision (Arvidsson *et al.*, 2000) found that participants reported that their feelings, thoughts and actions were confirmed during supervision. Similarly, a supervisee in a UK study (Hadfield, 2000) reported that, during CS, her skills and abilities as a practitioner were confirmed and affirmed. However, the approaches contributed towards confirmation and affirmation have remained elusive. Findings from the present study relating to the category 'agreeing with the supervisee' begin to clarify the ways in which supervisees' feelings, thoughts and actions can be confirmed by the supervisor during individual supervision.

In the following example, Megan agrees with Holly's realisation of how clinical realities differ from what she has read in professional texts. Megan discloses that she has had similar experiences. This particular approach may have had a reassuring, confidence-building influence.

Holly   Yeah, yeah, yeah. And when they keep talking about the group dynamics and that it's . . . I think I was expecting to be able to pick up a book, and they said you do this, this and this, but it's obviously like you say – it's not black and white.

Megan   That's it, Holly, that's exactly the way I thought it would happen. I would be able to pick up a book and read it and think that's the way I should do it.

(Case Site One, audio-recording with Megan and Holly, 11/02/00 p. 9)

In the following example, Nicola affirms David's opinion by agreeing with his comments on Ross and Jack.

David   There is one thing that you can say about Ross: one of his great strengths is his sensitivity.

Nicola   That's right.

David   I also found that about Jack over the years, and I've known him for years, that he is sensitive as well. He can be quite psychopathic in some of his decisions and he has to be because he is a senior manager.

Nicola   That's right.

David   Anything like that, he is sensitive.

Nicola   Yes.

(Case Site Two, audio-recording with David and Nicola, 31/10/00 p. 21)

Suggesting an option

CS has been promoted as an opportunity for practitioners to reflect on a broad range of concerns and sort out issues causing them difficulty (Docherty, 2000). Nevertheless, descriptions of the processes aimed at problem resolution are generally lacking in the supervision literature peculiar to nursing. One exception is that described by Rogers and Topping-Morris (1997). In their problem-focused model of CS, problem-solving strategies facilitate the identification of solutions to the clinical problems recognised by the supervisee. As an alternative to problem-focused supervision, Driscoll (2000b) encourages the adoption of a solution-focused approach. This approach incorporates ideas from solution-focused therapy (de Shazer, 1985). During supervision, the supervisor explores solutions, rather than attempts to analyse and resolve problems. Using this psychotherapy-based supervision model, the emphasis is on strengths, resources and exceptions to when problems are encountered. This approach would appear to have considerable benefits for healthcare professionals, particularly when consideration is given to the fact that opportunities to focus on strengths and affirmation of good work is so rare. Similarly, focusing on problems at every opportunity of CS may do little for either the supervisor's or supervisee's confidence.

However, clinical supervisors in each of the three teams in the current study used an alternative method. 'Suggesting an option' (Sloan, 2004) appeared to be an approach used by the majority of clinical supervisors.

Megan	And maybe introducing him to someone else. But working it out so that we have the best way to do that.
Lesley	Yes, I'll maybe say that to him. I'll see how he is. If he is feeling good, I'll maybe sort of say.
Megan	And maybe for him to go away and think about . . . does he wish to continue to see someone on a regular basis (*quietly spoken*).

(Case Site One, audio-recording with Megan and Lesley 21/10/99 p. 5)

Stephanie	Right. So I should maybe set up a meeting to discuss the possibility of her going to these places?
David	I think so, maybe presenting it to them as an option.
Stephanie	Right.
David	Maybe explain the type of people that use these facilities and let them decide then whether that's the sort of place they'd be happy with. You could even, if it was spoken about being arranged, arrange for (client N) and her sister and her mother or whoever to go up and have a look round the place first.
Stephanie	Right.

(Case Site Two, audio-recording with David and Stephanie, 10/12/99 p. 2)

| Daniel | The only other thing I'd ask you to consider, and we have spoken about it before, is would there in fact be scope for continuing this group in the |

(local area). Similar to (local village) on a Tuesday and (local village) on a Wednesday (*brief pause*). To me there's lots of benefits to that but from a case management benefit, if you like, the nursing assistants can see about eight patients in one go, if you like, and the patients would obviously benefit out of that as well hopefully in the group. So don't dismiss that.
(Case Site Three, audio-recording with Daniel and Claire, 29/08/00 p. 5)

When faced with a supervisee's uncertainty, the clinical supervisor would, more often than not, advise and offer guidance. This approach may have been endorsed by supervisors because, compared with facilitating another's discovery of solutions, it can be executed relatively quickly. Facilitating the supervisee's arrival at possible solutions would have demanded time, time which did not appear to be available. There was no evidence from any of the audio-recordings of supervisors following up on their suggestions and enquiring as to their usefulness, or otherwise, in subsequent sessions.

Giving feedback

'Giving feedback' (Sloan, 2004), while evident in all three teams, was more frequently observed in Case Site Three. In all three teams, the content of this feedback was positive.

The following example highlights a type of exchange that occurred infrequently in Megan's provision of CS.

Holly   I felt it went well and from a purely, I mean it is a, selfish point of view, because Gillian was late at it and I had to get on and present it. I feel sometimes they think the satellite groups are Gillian's because she's like the more dominant personality and I felt it gave me a chance to say this is what we're doing.

Megan   I thought you did really well, so I did, Holly . . . You know, we don't want to irritate people. We don't want to stand on folks' toes, and this is where we are and where you think, and I think you conducted it really well.
(Case Site One, audio-recording with Megan and Holly, 20/04/00 p. 7)

Holly would describe herself as being the lesser-known partner in comparison to Gillian in the context of their work on 'the satellite service' (Sloan, 2004). The situation highlighted above gave Holly the opportunity to present aspects of the service to managers and colleagues. Megan reinforced Holly's efforts by conveying positive feedback.

In the following example from Case Site Two, David offers Stephanie some praise for the progress she has made in her role.

Stephanie   Right. This lassie, she's discharged now and she's going to anxiety management. I've still to do that. Well, I've still to discharge her. She's been referred to the anxiety management. That's them.

David   That's good because the last time we were talking you got a lot of folk that you weren't sure what the actual direction you were going with was.
Stephanie   Aye, I'm getting to know what I'm doing with folk now.
David   Aye, you're becoming more focused. You know where you're taking them. You're planning to do things with them and then to discharge them. That's good. That's sometimes the hardest thing because when you come out here sometimes you just get these folk who you wonder what you're supposed to be doing and you can wander about for a wee while but that's good. You seem to know what you're going to be doing with them all.   *

(Case Site Two, audio-recording with David and Stephanie, 22/11/99 p. 18)

There were many instances from audio-recordings where Daniel would praise Claire's work. In the following examples, Daniel praised Claire's contribution to the team and her ability to manage her caseload.

Daniel   Well, maybe so, Claire, but I wouldn't underestimate the part you are playing in the fact that there's no conflict. And that's from what I'm seeing through there and at meetings as well and my own involvement with you.

(Case Site Three, audio-recording with Daniel and Claire, 22/02/00 p. 17)

Daniel   Right, OK (*brief pause*). See, by your very nature, Claire, you're a worker, quite simply you're a worker, you have a high caseload, you manage those caseloads and, I mean, I applaud that.

(Case Site Three, audio-recording with Daniel and Claire, 27/06/00 p. 6)

The particular role of 'giving feedback' in the context of CS has so far not received a great deal of attention in the nursing literature. Tapp and Wright (1996) describe the role of feedback in the context of live supervision during family therapy. In this setting, feedback is immediate and can increase the student's repertoire of interventions. It has been suggested that timely feedback in a supportive supervisory relationship can enhance the acquisition of professional knowledge and skills and lead to the development of valid and accurate self-evaluation (Farnill *et al.*, 1997). Moreover, there is a useful sequence to follow when providing feedback. Farnill *et al.* (1997) argue that factors shown to improve the efficacy of feedback include timely feedback, giving feedback in a climate of trust, specific and objective feedback, encourage self-evaluation first and then positive feedback followed by negative feedback. In the present study, as illustrated in the preceding examples, 'giving feedback' appeared to emanate from the clinical supervisors' managerial role.

Catalytic interventions

Secondary analysis using Heron's analytic framework illuminated three dominant categories of intervention common to all three teams. Catalytic, informative and supportive interventions were evident in all of the clinical supervisors' provision of supervision. Prescriptive interventions were observed to a lesser extent. Examples of cathartic and confronting interventions were almost negligible.

Catalytic interventions included the open and closed questions that were illuminated in the category 'seeking information'. Clinical supervisors in all three sites were observed to deliver mainly closed questions; open, explorative type questions were infrequent. The excessive use of closed questions and the limited delivery of open questions allowed each of the clinical supervisors to set parameters for supervisees' answers. Consequently, they limited the extent of the supervisees' exploration and discovery of new meaning. This finding corresponds with how the clinical supervisor's agenda had a strong influence over discussions during supervision. Furthermore, it illuminates how interactions during supervision limited the exploration of the complexities of everyday clinical practice, which contradicted findings relating to 'the stimuli for what is discussed during clinical supervision'. The lack of delivery of open, explorative questions, for example, reduced the likelihood of reaching any resolution to issues that emerged in the subcategories 'uncertainty' and 'problems' (Sloan, 2004). Since the section 'seeking information' illustrates this style of questioning, further examples are not required.

Empathic divining

The helping approach, labelled by Heron (1989, p. 101) as 'empathic divining', while not frequently observed, was delivered in Case Site One by Megan, and by Nicola in Case Site Two. It appeared to be used when the supervisee either expressed heightened feelings of distress or when talking about a difficult experience, for example Nicola demonstrated this approach when David described caring for a friend (see below) and when talking about a colleague returning following a long absence.

David	It was difficult for me emotionally I suppose because I like her a lot.
Nicola	Yes.
David	And she was wrecked and (Jean's husband) was wrecked as well.
Nicola	Yes.
David	Because they were thinking I was so calm and reassuring and I was (*laughing*).
Nicola	You were falling apart; I know, I know.
	(Case Site Two, audio-recording with David and Nicola, 31/10/00 p. 11)

Megan is able to pick up on the emotions lurking beneath what Gillian is saying in the following example.

| Gillian | (*sounding emotional*) Well, I was just, again it's probably because maybe I should have been assertive enough on the actual day and said, 'Well, does |

everybody feel that way', you know? But it was all made into a big joke, you know what I mean, and I let it be made into a big joke probably with my own defence mechanism, and it was all very much ... like, 'Here's Gillian and let's put this poster up and have a wee ticked box in it and Gillian could tick the box and that will make her happy', but it just didn't (*sounding tearful*).

Megan   You felt quite hurt by it all.
         (Megan and Gillian, audio-recording, 28/09/00 p. 15)

It has been suggested that the clinical supervisor's empathic understanding can contribute to the nurse's growth and learning (Trainor, 1978). When empathic divining was delivered in the present study, it would appear that at these times the clinical supervisor became alert to important events experienced by the supervisee. During these interactions, supervisors appeared to connect with the supervisees' feelings. In the example above from Case Site Two, Nicola is able to read between David's words and convey her empathy with the use of metaphor.

Informative interventions

Findings relating to informative interventions have been presented previously when discussing the category 'information-giving' and do not require further coverage.

Supportive interventions

One of the many alleged benefits of CS is that it is supportive (Wray *et al.*, 1998; Wilkin, 1999; Claveirole and Mathers, 2003). Despite the supportive aspect of CS having been evaluated in several studies (Butterworth *et al.*, 1997; Nicklin, 1997b; Teasdale *et al.*, 1998), the nature of supportive interactions has not been clarified. Findings presented previously relevant to the categories 'agreeing with the supervisee' and 'giving feedback' converge with supportive interventions, as described by Heron (1989).

A finding common to all three teams was the dominant feature of validation (positive feedback, praise, affirmation). Though much less frequent, there were examples of the clinical supervisors doing things for and giving things to the supervisee. A finding particular to Case Site One was touching; on a small number of occasions, Megan demonstrated her support by putting her arm around the supervisee's shoulder. The majority of supervisees valued these supportive approaches.

According to Heron (1989, p. 122), a validating intervention can also aim to celebrate the worth and value, the unique contribution, of the person. As the following example illustrates, validation is the sharing of a direct positive message.

Megan   I like the format you've got, you know, for recording and keeping an eye on, like from a personal point of view.

Holly   Well, I felt that all of this was so new, like forward planning and it was (team member) who'd used this and I thought it was really, really good.

Megan   I think so as well.

Holly   So I've borrowed it off her . . .

Megan   I think it's good. I think it's a great format.

Holly   Yeah. I've got like the dates that they started, when they need reviewing and that; so I find it's working.

Megan   And it will be quicker access for you to look at.

(Case Site One, audio-recording with Megan and Holly, 11/02/00 p. 5)

Nevertheless, many of the supportive exchanges appeared to emerge from clinical supervisors' managerial position, for example during supervision a supervisee would request some time off and the supervisor would oblige. This finding illuminates further the diverse ways in which managerial roles can encroach on CS.

Prescriptive interventions

Approaches that could be categorised as prescriptive interventions were much less frequently observed in all three sites. The approach described as 'suggesting an option' (Sloan, 2004) captured some examples of prescriptive interventions; however, there were others.

David delivered prescriptive interventions when Nicola discussed an issue she was uncertain about what to do about. For example, Nicola took two clinical issues to supervision and expressed her uncertainty about what to do about them. Following some questioning, David offered her suggestions. David took a similar approach when Nicola discussed issues that concerned her about her SN. In the following example, David delivers a 'benevolent directive intervention' (Heron, 1989, p. 35), suggesting how Nicola might communicate with her SN.

David   Maybe that's something else down the line. Like, 'OK, (team colleague), you know the assertiveness thing, that's working; we maybe need to look at how you pace your work.'

Nicola   Yes.

David   'How you pace what you're doing.'

Nicola   Yes, right.

David   'And we could have a look at that.'

Nicola   Yeah, yeah.

(Case Site Two, audio-recording with David and Nicola, 26/06/00 p. 30)

Heron (1989) suggests that prescriptive interventions usually refer to behaviour that was outside of the client–helper relationship. Nevertheless, there were examples of clinical supervisors guiding the supervisee about what to do during sessions including using the client list, where to sit and what to discuss. The following excerpts from Case Site One capture this sort of intervention.

Megan   So just run through the folk that are actually there.
(Case Site One, audio-recording with Megan and Gillian, 28/09/00 p. 1)

Megan   Just go through those you feel you need to speak about because I know you've got quite a few folk.
(Case Site One, audio-recording with Megan and Gillian, 16/10/00 p. 1)

Confronting interventions

Confronting interventions were almost negligible. Minimal reference was made to these types of intervention during interviews, and there was only one example observed from the audio-recordings of supervision. This type of intervention has not received a great deal of attention in the nursing literature pertaining to CS. Cutcliffe and Epling (1997, p. 175) describe confronting interventions as 'a gift with the capacity to enhance understanding and insight, rather than highlighting negative aspects of the individual'. Nevertheless, it would appear that confrontation is the category of intervention that some nurses find the most difficult to deliver (Burnard and Morrison, 1988; Morrison and Burnard, 1989). In the context of CS, where there is the possibility of the clinical supervisor hearing about practices that are not appropriate, confronting interventions may be useful. Similarly, when a supervisee is self-deprecating, the clinical supervisor could use confronting interventions to highlight strengths.

Cathartic interventions

The expression and discussion of feelings during CS is something that has been emphasised in the nursing literature (Faugier and Butterworth, 1994; Jones, 1999a; Proctor et al., 1999; Kipping, 2000). Moreover, dealing with clients' feelings is regarded as a core skill for mental health nursing (Faugier, 1996; Barker, 1999). In the present study, only a small minority of interviewees mentioned cathartic interventions. Furthermore, while some participants perceived that CS had a therapeutic quality, no interactions that focused on the exploration and processing of feelings were observed in any of the audio-recordings of supervision across all three teams.

Perhaps unpacking clients' feelings, particularly feelings of anger, fear and loss, and clinicians' reactions to this work would have taken too much effort and so it was avoided. Another possible reason suggested by Consedine (2000) is that mental health nurses are not yet ready to examine their clients' lives and their own responses to them. An effective supervisory relationship is necessary in order for these sorts of issues to be discussed in supervision. Furthermore, the relationship requires development before supervisees can feel safe enough to discuss this aspect of their clinical work. But, perhaps more importantly, clinicians must be working in particular ways, connecting with clients, in order to need this type of focus for supervision.

As described earlier, the practices of mental health nursing were criticised over 30 years ago as lacking in therapeutic intention (Altschul, 1972; Towell, 1975; Cormack, 1976). More recently, findings from research conducted by Gijbels (1995) illustrated the roles and skills that nurses performed were, it seemed, determined by organisational structures, ideologies, practices and policies over which nurses had, or exercised, little control. This resulted in unsystematic, unstructured, ad hoc, often interrupted and mainly reactive and controlling practices. Subsequently, it was concluded that these findings suggested that there had been very little forward movement in the therapeutic practices of mental health nurses over the past 25 years (Gijbels, 1995). From this perspective, it is perhaps understandable that mental health nurses in this study did not take advantage of the opportunity CS afforded for the exploration of the complexities of nurse–patient relations. It is therefore little wonder that CS was observed as being used for everything and anything.

Furthermore, this overview of mental health nursing practice might provide some explanation for the absence of particular interpersonal competence amongst clinical supervisors as observed during this investigation. If mental health nurses lack knowledge and skills in interpersonal relations in a clinical context, they cannot be expected to transfer them into CS.

Delivery of two interventions simultaneously

Six Category Intervention Analysis provides a catalogue of interventions from which a practitioner can choose. Heron (1989, p. 14) implies that during a helping exchange two categories of intervention could not be delivered simultaneously: 'The six categories are independent of each other in the sense that each has its relatively pure forms which cannot be reduced to the form of any other category.' Findings from Case Site Two and Three suggest that there can be a degree of amalgamation of intervention types. An intervention that crossed the boundaries of prescription and support emerged in Case Site Two since, during the delivery of the intervention, David's intention appeared to be both prescriptive (benevolent directive) and supportive (expressing concern). Similarly, in Case Site Three, Daniel delivered an intervention that appeared to be both informative and supportive.

Data from audio-recordings of supervision from Case Site Three provide numerous examples of an intervention that incorporated information-giving and being supportive. In these examples, as the clinical supervisor provided information he also conveyed a supportive stance towards Claire. In the example that follows, Claire has been describing a difficulty she had experienced because of her having a different opinion from the consultant psychiatrist.

Daniel   I agree with you, Claire, and certainly it's a common thing for a CPN to do where you go out, you assess, you see a person's depressed and you ask the GP to consider medication.

Claire   Yes.

Daniel   And I think that's fine and I've done that a hundred times, and the GP will informally, well no formally, say, 'What do you think I should give him?'

Claire   Well, I don't see any harm in saying what I think because there's an element of anxiety: 'What about an antidepressant with anxiolytic properties? How do you feel about that?' Because the GP then is perfectly entitled to say, 'Well, I don't think that's warranted' or 'Well, we'll go with that.' They will then decide which is the appropriate one or if there are no anxiety features in this, then it seems to be a straight depression. I think that's perfectly reasonable.

Daniel   Yeah, absolutely, and the bottom line of all this, Claire, is that a doctor has the responsibility to write the prescription.

Claire   Exactly.

Daniel   And whether he consults this one, that one or the next one, he puts pen to paper here and takes responsibility for doing that.

(Case Site Three, audio-recording with Daniel and Claire, 29/08/00 pp. 11–12)

These examples illuminate an intervention that incorporated a supportive element with another intention. This finding appears to provide some support for Morrison *et al.*'s (1991) investigation of the validity of the Six Category Intervention Analysis framework. Findings from Morrison *et al.*'s (1991) research provided little support for the division of authoritative and facilitative skills as described by Heron (1989). This new analysis, according to Morrison *et al.* (1991), suggests a different set of relationships: prescriptive and informative interventions are grouped together; confronting, cathartic and catalytic interventions are grouped together. Supportive interventions underpin both these groups. Findings from this study would appear to suggest that Heron's analytic framework requires some amendment.

Catalytic degenerate interventions

In addition to the six helpful categories of intervention, Heron (1989) describes degenerate and perverted interventions. Perverted interventions are deliberately malicious. The helper, when using this type of intervention, intends to do harm to the client. Their core purpose is to damage people. There was no evidence of perverted interventions in any of the teams participating in this research.

Degenerate interventions tend to be misguided helping and the result of the helper's lack of awareness, experience or training (Heron, 1989). There are four basic kinds: unsolicited, manipulative, compulsive and unskilled. In the present study, the degenerate interventions were mainly unsolicited and unskilled. Degenerate interventions were more evident where supervisees regarded the supervision they received as unhelpful, for example Case Site One. Nonetheless, degenerate interventions were also observed in Case Site Two and Three, where supervisees were more positive and satisfied with their experiences of supervision.

Catalytic degenerate interventions were observed in all three teams and emerged as the unskilled delivery of open and closed questions. As stated before, this limited the opportunities made available to supervisees to explore their clinical work. This finding appears to support the findings of earlier research (Burnard and Morrison, 1988, 1991; Morrison and Burnard, 1989; Ashmore and Banks, 1997), in whose investigations both student nurses and trained nursing staff perceived themselves as being weak in using catalytic interventions. In addition to the lack of open questions in the present study, there was an expectation that many of the issues could be covered during a relatively short period of time. Thus, clinical supervisors exerted control over the extent of discussions.

Cathartic degenerate interventions

Cathartic degenerate interventions and prescriptive degenerate interventions were observed in two of the teams. In Case Site One and Two, examples of cathartic degenerate interventions were illuminated. Despite strong emotions being expressed, there appeared to be avoidance of any exploration of, and not giving permission for, the expression of supervisees' feelings.

Supervisees from Case Site One commented that Megan never explored their feelings, which is evident from the audio-recordings. The following example illustrates an issue that was discussed during several sessions between Gillian and Megan. Gillian had been having a difficult time with a colleague, had received negative comments over a period of time and as a result felt stressed and was often emotional (sounding tearful) during supervision. At these times, while Megan gave her perspective on the situation, it would appear that she failed to acknowledge Gillian's distress or give permission to express her feelings. This seems contrary to the points Megan emphasises during her interview, particularly the emphasis placed on discussing staff relations and tending to the emotional well-being of her staff during CS.

Gillian   Right . . . and the only other thing I just . . . had wanted to bring up was
              remember, you know, it probably seems . . . it seems like a dim and distant
              past now but it really annoyed me at the time and kind of really plagued
              my mind for a wee while after it. If you remember at the management day
              . . . in the morning – and I've probably covered it – well, but I felt quite per-
              sonally attacked by somebody there . . . when they were talking about

attendances. We were talking about attendance for the flexible day service and again I had mentioned, I'd said to you before, that I'd had a comment from someone that I was a control freak and, you know, I was wanting everything, you know, done in certain ways and I was into these standards and audits and having protocols and everything like that and I was a control freak, and I had already said to you that I was kind of worried that that was the view of the staff about me, but the time that I was kind of acting up on your absence on holiday there didn't seem to be any problem and we seemed to work well as a team and everything was OK and I certainly didn't feel any animosity towards me, but just at the management day and it was the same person and it came across again and it was like (*brief pause*) this person was . . . acting as a spokesperson for the whole team when she said, 'Would you just shut up about your ticked boxes?' and 'Nobody's interested in that', and, you know, 'You're annoying the living daylights out of everybody and just everybody feels the same and nobody's got the guts to tell you', or something along those lines. I can't remember the exact words, but it was very much attacking anyway, although it was done with humour in the background, and it was, you know, 'Everybody feels the same about these ticked boxes and nobody's got the heart to tell you; you'll just need to give it a rest' kind of thing, and I felt so attacked and so insulted really in front of the whole team. I just didn't feel it was the place (*brief pause*). If that person had had a problem with that or if any of the team had had a problem with that, I didn't feel the management day was the place to personally attack me about it, and I don't know whether she had been a spokesperson for everybody else and that was the general feeling or whether she was just presuming that everybody felt the same way as she did. I really don't know, but I felt quite attacked and I felt quite isolated because, although there was humour behind it, I felt really quite hurt for the whole thing and . . .

Megan   Do you still feel like that?

Gillian   (*sounding emotional, tearful*) I meant to speak to the person individually and then . . .

Megan   I never recognised . . . it as being like that, Gillian . . . you know.

Gillian   I don't think, I mean I know the person and I have a good, I mean we have a good, relationship generally, aye. I know her manner is attacking and she can be difficult to take, normally if it's one to one and she says something to me then you know I can give as good as I get or I'll say to her, 'Well, I don't feel that', or 'I feel differently', or I can be quite assertive.

Megan   Yes.

Gillian   But it was when it was the whole team, you know, yourself, (consultant psychiatrist), everybody there, (team colleague), everybody was there and it was such a direct, attacking comment I just felt it was really . . .

Megan   But did you feel that the rest of the team were sort of, kind of . . .

Gillian   Well, everybody else just was silent really – do you know what I mean? Everybody else just – I mean – we were talking about the attendance for the flexible day service so the conversation just kind of carried on. I know . . . I took it very personally and probably nobody realised that but the conversation basically just carried on about how will we keep the attendance for the flexible day service because after she made that comment it just moved on to 'Well, how are we going to do it then?' and then it just was kind of carried on that way but . . .

Megan   You took it quite personally.

(Case Site One, audio-recording with Megan and Gillian, 28/09/00 p. 13)

This is surprising for a number of additional reasons. First, there was approval and an acknowledgement from participants that feelings were expressed during CS. Second, CS was thought to have a therapeutic purpose in these teams. Third, it is understood that CS provides an opportunity for the super-visee to make sense of feelings provoked by their clinical work (Jones, 1999b; Kipping, 2000; Odling et al., 2001). Finally, dealing with patients' feelings is regarded as an aspect of mental health nursing (Faugier, 1996).

Clinical supervisors in the present study may have avoided discussing feelings for the same reasons that prevented them from asking open, explorative questions. The time restrictions resulting from 'the routine' may have limited supervisors from focusing on feelings. It is acknowledged that the expression and processing of feelings takes time and the person expressing the feelings determines the pace and depth of exploration (Heron, 1989). On the other hand, clinical supervisors may have believed that it was too difficult to manage the strong feelings being expressed by supervisees, that is the sheer effort was too demanding.

Prescriptive degenerate interventions

Prescriptive degenerate interventions were observed in Case Site One and Three. In Case Site One, Megan demonstrated an unsolicited intervention by 'interfering take-over' (Heron, 1989, p. 191) where she would tell the supervisee that she would do things without negotiation. In Case Site Three, there appeared to be a perception shared amongst participants that CS provided an opportunity for the supervisee to look at alternatives and discover their own answers. Daniel explained that he wouldn't give answers and specific guidance to Claire – he saw little value in this and mentioned something about this approach stunting Claire's growth. Yet, from the audio-recordings, there were many examples of Daniel providing answers. These types of intervention were both unskilled (Daniel did something contrary to his description of what he did) and unsolicited (supervisees wanted to identify their own solutions to problems). In the following example, Daniel advises Claire on aspects of caseload manage-ment. He suggests that she make use of the team's nursing assistants.

Daniel   Yeah. The other thing I would say to you about (local village) in particular is that . . . OK designate Friday as your (local village) day so to speak . . . but remember that the nursing assistants, well (team colleague), goes up to (local village).

Claire   That's right.

Daniel   And if something crops up on a Monday or whatever and you think, 'Well, do I actually need to go away to (local village)?' No, ask the nursing assistant –

Claire   Yeah, yeah?

Daniel   – if she would pop in.

(Case Site Three, audio-recording with Daniel and Claire, 29/08/00 p. 16)

It is perhaps peculiar that Daniel, an experienced mental health nurse who had undergone further training in counselling, described his approach in supervision in a way that contradicted what was observed during audio-recordings of supervision. One explanation relates to the possibility of subject bias where Daniel described his approach in a way that he thought would be most acceptable. However, the researcher did not present an ideal format for supervision or express expectations for the delivery of CS. It is possible that other aspects of the team influenced the supervisor's delivery of CS. As high-lighted earlier, aspects of 'the routine' may have limited the time available for supervisors to facilitate supervisees towards their own solutions.

It is acknowledged by Driscoll (2000a) that providing answers may not be an effective strategy during CS. While there may well be times when some form of direction is required, supervisees may quickly realise that by asking the right questions they can persuade the supervisor to provide them with answers. Giving answers is quicker and easier than encouraging the supervisee towards discovering their own solutions. Nevertheless, this can 'lead to the supervisee becoming dependent on the supervisor' (Driscoll, 2000a, p. 130).

Comparisons with previous research using Heron's framework

The results of this study relating to Heron's framework bear some similarities with earlier work conducted by Burnard and Morrison (1988, 1991) and Morrison and Burnard (1989) (Table 7.1), as described in Chapter 4.

Findings derived from observation of CS using audio-recordings have some similarities with earlier work, which used a self-report method, particularly the work of Burnard and Morrison (1988, 1991) and Morrison and Burnard (1989). When mental health nurses' interactions were observed during individual CS, there was minimal evidence of either cathartic or confronting interventions. While there were numerous examples of catalytic interventions, particularly closed questions, generally the level of interpersonal skill in this intervention category was limited. The current study is also consistent with findings from Ashmore and Banks' (1997) investigation. Findings from the present study illustrate that mental health nurses delivered more facilitative interventions (catalytic and supportive).

OBJECTIVE 5

To explore how these interactions influence the content of supervision.

Table 7.1 Rank order of Six Category Intervention Analysis

Research Study	Ranking of Interventions					
Burnard and Morrison (1988, 1989, 1991)	Supportive	Informative	Prescriptive	Catalytic	Cathartic	Confronting
Ashmore and Banks (1997)	Supportive	Prescriptive	Cathartic	Informative	Catalytic	Confronting
Present study	Catalytic	Informative	Supportive	Prescriptive	Cathartic	Confronting

The results of the present study relating to this objective have been presented under Objective 1 and Objective 4 and do not require further elaboration.

OBJECTIVE 6

To illuminate the changes, resulting from supervision, as reported by participants.

It was anticipated that data emerging from individual in-depth interviews, audio-recordings of supervision and critical incident journals would illuminate changes, which may have been influenced by participants' engagement in CS. Consequently, changes are based on participants' self-reporting and observation of supervision sessions over a 12- to 18-month duration.

Case Site One

Findings from Case Site One suggest that the majority of participants did not acknowledge any positive changes resulting from their participation in CS. On the contrary, there was general acknowledgement that their participation in supervision had been detrimental. Supervisees commented that the negative feelings they had taken to supervision had been exacerbated as a result of unhelpful aspects. The majority of supervisees reported that their experience of supervision had been negative.

CS, according to Cotton (2001), has been promoted as inevitable, unproblematic, natural and desirable for nurses and nursing. For nurses not to want to participate in CS is seen as atypical, inconceivable, unprofessional and absurd. Yet, findings from recent research have indicated that engaging in CS can be quite a negative experience for some nurses. Teasdale et al. (1998) report that 17% of their sample had negative experiences. Participants in Draper et al.'s (1999) study became more negative about whether CS led to improved practice or enhanced professional practice. At the end of the project, less than half the participants felt CS would help them deal with difficult situations. During a telephone survey of practice nurses' views (Pateman, 2001), CS was equated with an invasion of clinical privacy, seen as a threat and generally negative. In the absence of positive changes, resulting from negative experiences, supervisees from Case Site One either looked for alternative means of support or hoped for something better to come along.

Case Site Two

Supervisees' opinions on CS in Case Site Two and Three were more favourable. Consequently, there was some acknowledgement of the positive changes they experienced. In Case Site Two, the changes that may have been influenced by discussions during CS emerged in the main categories: 'managing the caseload', 'professional development' and 'it's a therapeutic thing' (Sloan, 2004). A theme common to each of these categories, which is consistent with earlier work, was the reported increase in self-confidence.

Confidence-building was reported as one of the areas discussed during CS in Butterworth et al.'s (1998b) study. This appears to be reflective of a general opinion suggesting that CS is all about developing confidence (Cutcliffe and Proctor, 1998; Jones and Bennett, 1998; Wilson, 1999). Following a group experience of CS, supervisees reported an increase in their self-confidence (Dunn et al., 1999). In Case Site Two, there was some acknowledgement by both supervisees and clinical supervisors that their confidence had benefited from their experiences of supervision.

I feel I'm on top of my caseload just now and I was going through everybody and I knew exactly what I was doing with them and it was an opportunity to sort of establish that . . . and he could see that and he fed that back that things had been going all right for a while.
(Case Site Two, interview with Stephanie, supervisee, 23/03/01 p. 6)

I would like to think that you would notice that Nicola was becoming more confident about what she was doing . . . sometimes she does question herself . . . so you would like to see her own confidence improving.
(Case Site Two, interview with David, supervisor, 01/03/99 p. 15)

I think it enhances my clinical work in that it gives me more confidence.
(Case Site Two, interview with Nicola, supervisee and supervisor, 11/02/99 p. 10)

I suppose it kind of boosts your own, and it feels good to know you've helped someone, I suppose, in a way that you've been of some use, you know; that boosts your own confidence.
(Case Site Two, interview with Sarah, supervisor and supervisee, 11/03/99 p. 20)

8 Conclusion

INTRODUCTION

The aim of this study was to explore and describe the content of, processes within and changes resulting from the practice of CS by mental health nurses working in an NHS Primary Care Trust. The stimulus for the study was an awareness of the apparent broad scope for CS and the dearth of research relating to this area at the commencement of the study, as presented in Chapter 2. At the outset of the study, four key questions pertaining to the NHS Primary Care Trust were raised:

1. What is the content of individual CS for mental health nurses?
2. How do the interactions between clinical supervisor and supervisee during supervision sessions influence its content?
3. How do the organisational factors for CS affect the supervisory process?
4. What changes are reported from this experience of individual CS?

This chapter, in concluding the report of the study, reflects on the extent to which these questions have been answered. It does this by highlighting the major insights gained by the study while acknowledging its limitations and discusses the contribution the study makes to knowledge.

MAJOR INSIGHTS GAINED FROM THE STUDY

THE CONTENT OF CLINICAL SUPERVISION

The findings from this study indicate that CS had a broad scope. Managerial agendas appeared to have had considerable emphasis during CS. Performance appraisal, professional development plans, service developments, staff relations and off-duty were frequently incorporated into discussions. Supervision was regarded as a stress-relieving resource in all three teams and perceived as having a particular therapeutic purpose in two of the teams. Ultimately, there was widespread endorsement by all participants that anything and everything could be discussed during CS. Supervisees' clinical issues were observed to be less of a priority. There appeared to be a powerful risk-management agenda underpinning 'safe practice' and 'doing the right thing' (Sloan, 2004), both of which were recurring themes that stimulated discussions during supervision. Consequently, these discussions, which were heavily influenced by clinical supervisors, came across as pertaining to caseload management. At these times, it was observed that supervisees would provide an update of many patients in a short period of time.

INTERPERSONAL INTERACTIONS AND THEIR INFLUENCE ON CONTENT

In Chapters 1 and 2, attention was drawn to some of the theoretical and conceptual complexities pertaining to CS. It was argued that the literature suggests that CS has a broad purpose in nursing, and it would appear that conceptual ambiguities influence the ways in which it is practised. Findings from this study suggest that CS is not straightforward to practise.

Observation of clinical supervisors and supervisees engaging in CS illuminated frequently recurring modes of interpersonal interaction. The dominant supervisors' approaches observed during interpersonal interactions between clinical supervisors and supervisees that emerged from open thematic analysis included 'seeking information', 'information-giving', 'agreeing with the supervisee', 'suggesting an option' and 'giving feedback' (Sloan, 2004). These approaches corresponded with findings that emerged from secondary analysis using Heron's (1989) Six Category Intervention Analysis. Catalytic, informative, supportive and prescriptive interventions were the most frequently observed categories in this study.

Deeper analysis of supervisor–supervisee interactions (Sloan, 2004) illuminated the essence of these types of intervention. 'Seeking information' (catalytic interventions) was monopolised with closed questions; open exploratory questions were rarely observed. The nature of 'information-giving' (informative interventions) generally related to supervisors sharing factual information concerning clients, their thoughts and opinions about clients and operational aspects relating to particular Trust procedures. 'Agreeing with the supervisee' and 'giving feedback' (supportive interventions) begin to clarify ways in which a supervisee's feelings, thoughts and actions can be confirmed during CS. 'Suggesting an option' (prescriptive interventions) was delivered when the supervisee appeared uncertain of what to do. Furthermore, clinical supervisors were prescriptive when telling the supervisee what to do during sessions, for example using the client list, where to sit and what to discuss.

The nature of these interventions illuminated the authoritative position of the clinical supervisor/manager in the supervisory relationship. In asking closed questions, clinical supervisors limited the scope of CS to filling the gaps in their knowledge. Informative interventions facilitated the sharing of mainly managerial issues, and prescriptive interventions enabled managers to tell supervisees what to do within and outwith CS. Similarly, supportive interventions appeared to emanate from the clinical supervisor's managerial role.

However, the uncovering of degenerate interventions in all supervision pairs in the present study illuminates further difficulty in practising CS. Catalytic degenerate interventions were observed in all three teams and emerged as the unskilled delivery of open and closed questions. In Case Site One and Two, examples of cathartic degenerate interventions emerged. Finally, prescriptive degenerate interventions were observed in Case Site One and Three. Supervisees working in Case Site One felt that it was the lack of knowledge and understanding that contributed to their supervisors' delivery of unhelpful CS. However, the emergence of other categories from open thematic analysis suggests that the organisational context might also have contributed to the ways in which clinical supervisors practised CS.

ORGANISATIONAL FACTORS AND THEIR INFLUENCE ON THE SUPERVISORY PROCESS

In the present study, three categories – 'the stimuli for what is discussed during clinical supervision', 'preparation for clinical supervision' and 'the routine' (Sloan, 2004) – emerged, illuminating the organisational provision for CS and its influence on supervisory processes.

The stimuli for what is discussed during clinical supervision

'Problems' and 'doing the right thing' were recurring themes for the category of 'the stimuli for what is discussed during clinical supervision' (Sloan, 2004). The majority of participants regarded CS as an opportunity to deal with any problems that a supervisee might experience. It was thought that dealing with 'problems' would ensure supervisees were 'doing the right thing'. 'Doing the right thing' appeared to have some connection with ensuring 'safe practice'. The emphasis placed on 'safety', however, appeared to reduce the opportunities for exploration and reflection of clinical practice regardless of whether it was either good or bad. There were limited opportunities for facilitating supervisees' reflections on 'good enough' practices. With so much emphasis being placed on identifying and resolving problems, there appeared to be limited opportunity for nurses to reflect on their relations with patients or acknowledge and celebrate examples of good practice.

Preparation for clinical supervision

Participants in all three teams had limited preparation for their engagement in CS. The majority of participants relied on their own previous experiences of being a recipient of supervision to guide their own delivery. The provision of CS, at the commencement of the study, was confined to CMHTs and was hierarchical. Thus, supervisees in the present study received supervision from their managers, who in turn had received supervision from their managers.

There were a small number of participants who had undergone some form of formalised preparation for CS, a university-based module on CS as part-fulfilment for their degree. However, opportunities were not made available for SNs, who had completed the module, to utilise the knowledge and skills in the role of clinical supervisor. While the content of the supervision module may have increased these participants' ability to engage in supervision as supervisees, opportunities to develop as clinical supervisors were not offered.

Only one of the clinical supervisors in the study had completed the academic module. While he felt better prepared for the role as clinical supervisor, similar to the supervisees, the module had furnished him with a theoretical and conceptual knowledge and understanding of CS, which heightened his insight of the constraints of 'the routine'. Consequently, he attempted to challenge 'the routine'. Nevertheless, this level of preparation did not appear to prepare him for the complexities and challenges of providing CS in practice.

The routine

The organisational provision of CS presented under the category of 'the routine' was traced back to its initial inception. Present-day hierarchical arrangements resemble how CS was provided during its early years. Consequently, in all three teams there was a powerful managerial influence over participants' engagement in CS. 'The supervisor's agenda' subjugated supervisees' contribution towards the content of, and knowledge demonstrated during, CS. It would appear that, in fulfilling this dual role, the managerial aspect deskilled mental health nurses in terms of their interpersonal communication and awareness of the complex issues pertaining to clinical practice. This brings into question the suitability of a line manager to provide CS.

CHANGES REPORTED FROM THE EXPERIENCE OF INDIVIDUAL CLINICAL SUPERVISION

Supervisees from Case Site One were unable to identify any positive changes resulting from their experience of CS. On the contrary, these supervisees commented on the negative effects of participating in supervision. This situation would appear to have been influenced by both the organisational provision of CS and the clinical supervisor's lack of experience in supervision.

Findings from the remaining teams suggest that those participating in CS experienced changes at a personal level, usually by way of an increased self-confidence and self-esteem, reduced stress levels and generally feeling happier in themselves. Furthermore, CS was believed to have a positive influence on team morale. The contribution of CS on the professional development of individuals was also acknowledged. Some supervisees had noticed their development in working with particular clinical issues, for example elder abuse, ongoing academic development, meeting personal goals identified on Personal

individual teams afforded this concept. Where there was an emphasis on CS having some degree of therapeutic focus, there were expectations of a therapeutic outcome and some enhancement of the emotional well-being of the supervisee. While all the teams gave time for the discussion of patient-related issues, it was clear that this opportunity was confined to providing an update rather than a deeper exploration of nurses' relations with patients. Consequently, there did not appear to be an expectation of supervision influencing changes specific to patient care.

Through an investigation of CS, an opportunity was provided to elicit a degree of understanding of the nature of mental health nursing in a clinical context. In particular, the extent of mental health nurses' focus on their relationship with patients became apparent. It is evident from this study that mental health nurses talked about issues relating to the assessment of patients' mental health, discharge procedures, liaising with other professionals and medication during CS. At least during CS, mental health nurses did not explore issues relating to how they related with patients or the nursing contribution between assessment and discharge.

This investigation provided an opportunity to observe the interpersonal interactions between supervisors and their supervisees during CS. Consequently, it facilitated an exploration of mental health nurses' interpersonal competence, at least as observed during CS. The implication is that mental health nurses in the role of clinical supervisor appeared to be limited in their delivery of explorative questioning. Furthermore, there is an implication that these mental health nurses lacked an ability to focus on, and promote, the exploration of supervisees' reactions to their work.

Six Category Intervention Analysis is already recognised as a useful framework that mental health nurses can work from when interacting with patients (Chambers, 1990; Ashmore, 1999). Burnard (1985, 2002), in particular, supports its use in general nursing contexts. Findings from this study have illustrated its usefulness in analysing mental health nurses' interpersonal interactions in the context of CS; helpful and unhelpful interactions were captured using the framework. The implication for the framework is that it appears to be a suitable teaching resource to explore the interactional styles of mental health nurses. In addition, it may serve as a useful resource to expand mental health nurses' interpersonal skills.

Nurse education

This study has identified gaps in the practice of experienced mental health nurses, some of whom had undertaken further post-registration education. The implication is that the educational requirements of those participating in CS extend beyond the theory and skills pertaining to CS. It would appear that the inclusion of interpersonal relations, research awareness and evidence-based mental health nursing is required. However, this level of preparation may not be confined to mental health nurses but a requirement of nurses working in a wide range of clinical contexts.

Nursing research

This investigation has highlighted the relevance of using illuminative evaluation for a study focusing on phenomena such as the practice of individual CS in mental health nursing. The approach was flexible and comprehensive enough to illuminate the influence of the learning milieu on modifying the instructional system, by focusing on the performance of individual CS. This was further aided by a study design that incorporated analysing data from three case sites. The implication is that illuminative evaluation is worthy of consideration because of its ability to explore the learning milieu and how this affects innovations with an educational basis. Consequently, illuminative evaluation would appear to be a suitable method for the study of preceptorship, mentorship, critical companionship and reflective practice. It should be used cautiously, however, since it has the potential to create a substantial database requiring considerable time and effort for data analysis.

LIMITATIONS OF THE STUDY

RESEARCHER

One limitation was in respect of my capability to conduct an illuminative evaluation of CS that incorporated multiple triangulation. The data-collection methods produced a substantial amount of data. Furthermore, data from the interviews and audio-recordings were subjected to secondary analysis. Collecting, managing and analysing these data was challenging and required a great deal of concentrated effort and time. While these obstacles were surmounted and did not threaten the quality of the investigation, at times the sheer task of analysis seemed overwhelming.

PARTICIPANTS

Those participating in the study provided a wealth of information. All participants engaged in one or more interviews; clinical supervisors and supervisees also provided audio-recordings of their supervision and, in addition to this, supervisees provided CS session records and critical incident journals. Nonetheless, the work circumstances of certain individual participants changed during the study. Consequently, some participants had to withdraw from the study. However, a flexible approach was required in order to maintain some of the other participants' engagement in the research. Thus, some participants' engagement in CS may have changed as a result of the changes to their work circumstances.

STUDY DESIGN AND METHODS

Study site

The study was conducted in one NHS Primary Care Trust. Since there is no directly equivalent study or emergent data, it could be claimed that the findings of the study are confined to this single site. Nonetheless, as reported in Chapter 7, there are similarities to be found in the results from previous research. It is possible that the study site itself, in particular the three teams, shared similarities with other teams in mental health services situated within NHS Primary Care Trusts throughout the UK.

Critical incident journal

A further limitation relates to the data-collection methods. Despite having been provided with repeated explanations on how to complete their critical incident journals, participants provided descriptions of the interactions with their clinical supervisors instead of describing how CS impacted on their practice. While this did provide a further perspective on the supervisory relationship, it did not allow for description of the impact CS had on these nurses' clinical practice. Consequently, there was perhaps a paucity of data regarding changes influenced by supervision.

Audio-recording supervision sessions

The limitations of audio-recording supervision sessions must be acknowledged. Clinical supervisors and supervisees had control over when the recording device was switched on. It is possible that discussions pertinent to supervision took place both before the recording device had been switched on and after it had been turned off. Furthermore, it is possible that the clinical supervisor and supervisee discussed issues at other times during their day-to-day contact. This may have influenced what the supervisee had to say and how the supervisor responded and therefore the depth of discussions during sessions. When asked about this, participants denied that it took place. They stressed that the audio-recordings captured the full extent of discussions. This uncertainty could have been resolved by requesting supervisees to maintain a diary of the times they discussed issues with their supervisor outwith formalised CS. However, this would have been an additional demand on participants' time and not relevant to the specific focus of this study.

Six Category Intervention Analysis

Heron (1989) argues that verbal behaviour could be described in three different ways: verbatim, linguistic and intention. Based on verbatim, linguistic and context, I made assumptions with regards to what the clinical supervisor had intended and categorised each exchange accordingly, for example informative or supportive. Later, when I subjected my analysis to member checking, I sought verification of this categorisation from the clinical supervisors. This took place some time after these supervision sessions had been recorded. None of the clinical supervisors challenged my interpretation and felt that the categorisation of their exchanges was appropriate. Furthermore, I requested each of my academic supervisors to conduct an independent analysis to validate my interpretation. However, verification of clinical supervisors' intentions could have been sought earlier, for example as close to the supervision session as possible. This would have facilitated supervisors to state their own understanding of what their intentions had been rather than verifying the researcher's interpretation. On practical terms, this would have been complicated and more intrusive of participants' work routines.

While the framework facilitated the identification of degenerate interventions, supervisees in Case Site One reported unhelpful ways Megan delivered CS, which, while captured from thematic analysis, did not emerge under Heron's categories. Supervisees in Case Site One, for example, reported that Megan would often take discussions away from their issues and share personal information. Had this information not emerged during interviews, this style of interacting may have been interpreted as an informative intervention. The consideration of all data captured through multiple triangulation and returning to participants for member checking reduced the potential for misinterpretations.

Trustworthiness

To ensure the trustworthiness of data from the present study, a number of strategies were adopted. These included prolonged engagement, persistent observation, member checking and validation of data analysis by academic supervisors. Consequently, it is hoped that this study presents a rich, contextually relevant description of CS. Team descriptions, documents relevant to how CS has been endorsed in the site and other data derived from the study have contributed to this account. Nevertheless, the study was conducted in three teams within one site and, while data analysis and findings are recognised by their participants, they may not be credible to others. The transferability of these findings is open to question and dependent on the reader.

CONTRIBUTION TO KNOWLEDGE

CLINICAL SUPERVISION

While there has been a steady growth in the empirical-evidence and theoretical developments in CS, this study too makes a contribution to knowledge.

The study provides improved insight into the contextual factors influencing how its participants experience CS. It also sheds light on the complex nature of supervision, particularly how dual roles impact on what happens during sessions. Furthermore, the study illuminated how supervisory processes and, in particular, how supervisor behaviours influenced the content and subsequent changes emanating from supervision. Supervisor approaches that elicit information, provide information, are supportive and prescriptive were illuminated. In addition, unhelpful aspects of supervision were uncovered. The current study contributes to the understanding of how individual CS has been adopted by nurses working in mental health. However, findings may have some relevance to nurses working in other clinical areas and also the practice of CS by other healthcare practitioners, for example counselling, clinical psychology and psychotherapy.

NURSE EDUCATION

Findings from the study may too contribute to future educational programmes for those clinicians engaged in CS. Furthermore, findings may be useful to other educationally focused innovations, for example preceptorship, mentorship, critical companionship and reflective practice.

NURSING RESEARCH

Previous published research on CS has not used an illuminative-evaluation methodology. The contribution of using this approach to study CS has been acknowledged. Thus, this is a preliminary step towards further process-focused research. Moreover, the benefits in adopting audio-recordings in a study focusing on the interpersonal processes integral to CS have been recognised.

SIX CATEGORY INTERVENTION ANALYSIS

The current study also contributes to previous research concerning Heron's (1989) Six Category Intervention Analysis, particularly the work conducted by Burnard and Morrison (1988, 1991) and Ashmore and Banks (1997). This study used Heron's analytic framework to analyse supervisor behaviours during supervision sessions rather than, as in earlier work, asking participants to self-report using a rating scale. Findings from the study would suggest that Heron's framework requires some level of modification and further inquiry.

CONCLUSION

This study focused on the interpersonal interactions between the clinical supervisor and supervisee. It emerged that the context within which CS was provided had a significant influence on how it was experienced. Aspects of the instructional system, particularly a Trust document and module descriptor for a CS module, were unable to penetrate the rigid and inflexible provision of CS.

There was considerable expectation that mental health nurses, because of a recognition of the skills integral to mental health nursing, could assume the role of clinical supervisor with minimal formalised preparation. These clinical supervisors were expected to take on the demanding and complex role with no support structures or ongoing development. It emerged that when clinical supervisors also assumed a line-management function, because of dual-role incompatibilities, covert tensions impinged on the experience of CS.

These tensions were illuminated as the reciprocal interpersonal interactions between the clinical supervisor and supervisee were brought into focus. Secondary analysis confirmed findings from open thematic analysis. Not surprisingly, unhelpful exchanges were illuminated. While this study has uncovered a number of weaknesses in the process of CS and gaps in mental health nurses' level of competence in interpersonal relations, it has provided a basis for a more critical approach to this important element of professional development.

There are a number of important and pressing areas for the continuing development of CS in nursing. Further exploration and clarification about CS is required. On reflection, what a small number of the supervisees in this study needed from CS was similar to my own needs as a mental health nurse, a relationship, where time and skill facilitated the exploration of the interpersonal fusion between nurse and patient. If we return to my early experiences of CS as presented in Chapter 1, it was my own beliefs that were impacting on the care I provided. An exploration of this might have helped me 'unlock doors', discover my 'errors' and furnish me with the necessary insight in order to modify my presence and care delivery with these clients. If this opportunity is not made available during CS, where else is there for the complexities of one's clinical work to be explored?

It is also necessary to identify the particular skills and relationship formation necessary for effective supervision in nursing. My first clinical supervisor was kind, supportive and provided me with reassurance. Nonetheless, similar to the clinical supervisors in this study, instead of support and reassurance, exploration and stimulating challenge may have been more appropriate. At this point, Wilkin's words of wisdom are relevant:

It is essential that we view clinical supervision in a facilitative context as opposed to being somewhat of an imposition. Supervision should be an unshackling process – an opening of previously locked doors . . . It should not be an invasion of inner privacy but a much more tentative and empathic exercise. It should be non-threatening enough to ensure participation, yet challenging and stimulating enough to encourage exploration. (Wilkin, 1998, p. 202)

It would appear that while there are some transferable skills that nurses can use in their supervisory practice, the goals of supervision are very different from those of clinical nursing and require different skills. Training in CS should highlight the ways in which supervision and the clinical practice of nursing are similar and different. But training in CS has more important priorities and should focus on those approaches that facilitate learning, take cognisance of the interpersonal context of helping relationships and delineate clear boundaries of the supervisory relationship. This study provides substantial evidence to justify the need for such developments.

RECOMMENDATIONS

The recommendations to arise from this study are aimed at the future development of CS. It is important to reiterate that this study was conducted in one MHD of a Primary Care Trust in Scotland, and only the reader can determine the transferability of findings and relevance of these broad recommendations to their own area, after considering the description of the context and conduct of this study.

1. Based on the conceptual misunderstanding surrounding CS, there is a necessity to revisit its value in facilitating the therapeutic development and competence of the supervisee and consider the relevance of this to those nursing contexts within which CS is practised. Agreement on the precise purpose of the supervisory endeavour needs to be made. This should occur at a professional level with scholarly debate, the organisational context within which CS is practised and with those practitioners engaging in CS.
2. Training in CS should focus on those approaches that facilitate learning, take cognisance of the interpersonal context of helping relationships and delineate clear boundaries of the supervisory relationship.
3. Following on from the second recommendation, future CS research in nursing should investigate the approaches that are conducive to facilitating exploration of nurse–patient relations and related issues. The nature of CS provided by a clinical supervisor with no managerial responsibility over the supervisee should be explored. There is also scope to investigate CS, focusing on the therapeutic work of mental health nurses, particularly those in specialist positions. Similarly, this area of focus in other nursing specialties is necessary. Obviously, the conceptual models for CS require detailed exploration and evaluation.
4. A practitioner who has no line-management role over the supervisee should provide clinical supervision.
5. Trusts should explore the use of supervision networks and directories as a means of organising and advertising the availability of suitably qualified clinical supervisors.

6. CS should be guided by a conceptual framework that is consistent with that which underpins the supervisee's clinical practice.

7. Clinical supervisors' and supervisees' engagement in CS should be nurtured with ongoing training and support.

8. CS requires considerable investment. Trusts should strive for agreement amongst major stakeholders on the specific outcomes expected from practitioners engaging in CS so that its value can be evaluated.

9. Heron's analytic framework should be used to investigate nurses' interactions with patients in various clinical contexts. In addition to facilitating the discovery of nurses' interpersonal interactions with patients, this research would provide further opportunities to progress Heron's framework.

10. Multiple triangulation is recommended for research investigating interpersonal interactions. In particular, the use of across-method triangulation, which might include interviews and audio-recordings of interactions, provides a rich perspective.

Appendix 1 Community Health Care Trust

DISCUSSION PAPER ON CLINICAL SUPERVISION FOR NURSING WITHIN THE COMMUNITY HEALTH CARE TRUST

This discussion paper will address specific issues related to the implementation of clinical supervision.

An argument supporting the need for clinical supervision will be developed. From this, a working definition will form the basis of a useful framework. After the various models of delivery are detailed, the requisite characteristics of both supervisor and supervisee and the core rules for the process of clinical supervision within this Trust will be outlined.

It is anticipated that the discussion provoked by this document will lead to the implementation of effective clinical supervision in nursing Trust-wide. Ultimately, effective clinical supervision will lead to an improved quality of patient care.

1. CLINICAL SUPERVISION IN OTHER PROFESSIONS

1.1 Clinical supervision in social work, psychotherapy and counselling has been in existence for a number of years. However, within each of these helping professions, its focus has changed.

1.2 For example, in social work, clinical supervision was initially a purely educational process; yet, in a review in 1976, its function has developed into an administrative and supportive mechanism while retaining its educational role.

1.3 Similarly, a shifting emphasis is reported in psychotherapy. Within the auspices of psychoanalysis, clinical supervision was seen as therapy for the therapists (Schlessinger, 1966). However, today, supervision is moving towards an eclectic model focusing on the educational elements of the supervisory process. Its main purpose is the acquisition of therapeutic skills.

2. THE LACK OF CLINICAL SUPERVISION IN NURSING

2.1 The concept of clinical supervision has simultaneously excited and confused nurses in a manner reminiscent of the introduction of the nursing process.

2.2 The term 'clinical supervision' has created a degree of confusion in the minds of many. Often, it is automatically associated with a managerial relationship and in particular the negative misconceptions inherent in this. Platt-Koch (1986) suggests, for many nurses, 'supervision means observation by an administrative superior who inspects, directs, controls and evaluates the nurse's work'.

2.3 Another equally unfavourable misconception is when clinical supervision is seen solely as a support framework for nurses on the verge of burnout. The extent of stress, and indeed burnout, in nursing is well documented (Sadler, 1988; Mackinick and Mackinick, 1990; Boyle *et al.*, 1991; Williams, 1991) as are the consequences, for example absenteeism, leaving the profession and professional misconduct. However, it is equally well known that nurses have difficulty in recognising the telltale signs of such phenomena in themselves, or, indeed, offering a supportive role to their colleagues.

2.4 There are some pockets of good examples of clinical supervision throughout the United Kingdom. Unfortunately, the process is very often confined to clinical specialists or nursing's elite. In the past, according to Faugier and Butterworth (1994), an attitude existed that implied clinical supervision was for the favoured few.

2.5 Finally, nursing as an established occupation has existed since the 1820s without any formal system of clinical supervision. Why, then, is the need for this process appearing today?

2.6 Before addressing this question, it should be stated that, until quite recently, there has been no formal acknowledgement of the need for clinical supervision in nursing.

2.7 Following the Department of Health's (DoH, 1993) document *A Vision for the Future – The Nursing, Midwifery and Health Visiting Contribution to Health and Health Care* specifically targeting 'the vision', which describes clinical supervision as:

> A formal process of professional support and learning which enables individual practitioners to develop knowledge and competence, assume responsibility for their own practice and enhance consumer protection and safety of care in complex clinical situations.

the introduction of a formal model of clinical supervision for nursing and health visiting now seems inevitable.

3. THE NEED FOR CLINICAL SUPERVISION

3.1 The literature tends to consider clinical supervision as a good thing. If it were to be developed and formalised, this would be to the advantage of nursing and patient care. For example, Nicklin (1995) suggests that clinical supervision can lead to:

- improved patient care;
- improved staff performance;
- improved managerial performance;
- risk reduction, i.e. decrease the number of complaints, errors etc.

These assumptions seem to put forward clinical supervision as a panacea for many nursing dilemmas. Importantly, the evidence on which these assumptions are based requires further development.

3.2 There is recognition of the advances that have been occurring within nursing over the last 20 years. Nursing has moved from a traditional bureaucratic work style where status took precedence to a professional cognitive style where patient needs are cared for in an individualised and holistic way (Drummond, 1990). The Nursing Process, Conceptual Frameworks for Practice, Primary Nursing, Named Nursing, and of Educational Reforms (UKCC, 1986) have all contributed to this advancement.

3.3 Since 1984, there has been an increasing recognition of nurses' individual accountability for their actions under the UKCC Code of Professional Conduct (UKCC, 1990).

3.4 Clinical supervision can be utilised as a mechanism for socialisation where the neophyte, upon qualifying, may internalise the desired knowledge, approved behaviours and accepted attitudes that belong to the culture (Melia, 1987). In many ways, clinical supervision is an extension of the preceptorship experience students receive during their nurse education. PREP (UKCC, 1990) has acknowledged the importance of this experience by recommending newly qualified staff having a preceptor for an initial six-month period.

3.5 The source of nursing knowledge has moved away from being exclusively based on the ward to a more definite emphasis on the literature; the view in nursing now is that developments in practice arise from research and reflective practice, as opposed to the repetition of ritual and routine (Fowler, 1996a).

3.6 Further, a variety of policy statements and position papers (DoH, 1993, 1994b; UKCC, 1995; Faugier and Butterworth, 1994) support the need for clinical supervision.

3.7 Within nursing, there is also a growing acceptance that feelings of discouragement, emotional exhaustion and burnout can be minimised by clinical supervision (Firth, 1986).

4. WHAT IS CLINICAL SUPERVISION?

4.1 An exchange between practising professionals to enable the development of professional skills (Butterworth and Faugier, 1992)

A formal process of professional support and learning which enables individual practitioners to develop knowledge and competence, assume responsibility for their own practice and enhance consumer protection and safety of care in complex clinical situations. (DoH, 1993)

Both definitions emphasise the educational and quality-assurance functions of clinical supervision; however, because of its absence in the above definitions, the supportive function is overlooked.

4.2 Instead the following definition should also be considered:

> An interpersonal process where a skilled practitioner helps a less skilled/experienced practitioner to achieve professional abilities appropriate to his/her role. (Barber and Norman, 1987)

4.3 From the Community Health Care Trust Clinical Supervision Working Group, the following definition is offered:

> Clinical supervision is a dynamic process that provides opportunities for practising nurses to openly discuss with seniors, peers or other professional specialists, individually or in a group, all areas of clinical practice to establish, promote and maintain a high standard of care delivery and is an integral part of professional development.

4.4 Confusion may arise due to similarities with the previously sited definitions of clinical supervision and other resources, such as mentorship (Darling, 1984) and preceptorship (UKCC, 1990), which are often used as umbrella terms in the nursing literature.

4.5 The Department of Health's (DoH, 1993) document uses the term 'clinical supervision'. This may be the term of choice.

5. FRAMEWORK FOR SUPERVISION

5.1 Following a review of several frameworks, Proctor's three-function model of supervision would appear appropriate and applicable in the disparate nursing situations found within the Community Health Care Trust.

5.2 This model has three main functions:
- formative
- normative
- restorative.

5.3 The formative function is primarily concerned with developing skills and expanding the practitioner's knowledge base. This can be achieved by:
- reflective practice;
- exploration of interventions used by the nurse;
- exploration of the nurse–client relationship.

Its focus is educational.

5.4 The normative function assures quality by the ongoing assessment and evaluation of the standards of clinical practice. It has a managerial emphasis.

5.5 The restorative function and its supportive role attempts to alleviate the stress inherent within the sphere of nursing practice. Hawkins and Shohet

Appendix 2

INTERVIEW SCHEDULE – CLINICAL SUPERVISORS

- How is supervision organised between you and your supervisee? Frequency, who, when, where? Preparation, training, etc. What factors influence this? What influence do you have over this?

- What emphasis do you place on the provision of clinical supervision?

- What, in your opinion, is clinical supervision all about? What purpose does it serve?

- How would you explain how you conduct a supervision session to a complete stranger to the concept? If someone were watching you during a session, what would they notice about you?

- Can you recall a supervision session when the supervisee made particular use of the session? How did you contribute to this? Are there any other ways in which supervision is used?

- What supervisory behaviours/qualities/styles/skills you demonstrate are important? How would you describe your style of supervision? Can you give me any examples?

- What effects does supervision have on the supervisee? At a personal level? As a clinician? To the patient/client? Can you give me any examples?

- What, if anything, would you change in the supervision you provide?

- What, if any, are the difficulties in providing supervision? Are there particular aspects you find difficult? Tell me about any aspect of supervision that you feel is unhelpful?

- How do you evaluate the supervision you provide?

- Are there any other aspects of the clinical supervision in your area which you feel would be helpful for me to know about?

Appendix 3

CLINICAL SUPERVISION SESSION RECORD

Supervisee _____   Session type _____

Supervisor _____   Date _____

Duration _____   No of CS sessions _____   Total time _____

Agenda for CS
Record of issues discussed
Actions following session

Date and time of next session _____

REFERENCES

Abel-Smith, B. (1960) *A History of the Nursing Profession*, Heinemann, London.

Adams, T. (1991) Clinical supervision: psychiatric students. *Nursing Standard*, 5 (26), pp. 29–31.

Adcock, L. (1999) Clinical supervision in practice. *Journal of Community Nursing*, 13 (5), pp. 4–6.

Alexis, O. (2002) Securing the future of the NHS: developing and supporting staff nurses. *Nursing Management*, 9 (2), pp. 15–17.

Allan, G.J., Szollos, S.J., Williams, B.E. (1986) Doctoral students' comparative evaluations of best and worst psychotherapy supervision. *Professional Psychology: Research and Practice*, 17 (7), pp. 91–99.

Altschul, A.T. (1972) *Patient-Nurse Interaction: A Study of Interaction Patterns in Acute Psychiatric Wards*, Churchill Livingstone, London.

Anderson, C., Dorsay, J.P. (1998) Viewing rehabilitation nursing like a 'magic eye' picture: clinical supervision can sharpen the focus. *Rehabilitation Nursing*, 23 (6), pp. 305–308.

Arvidsson, B., Lofgren, H., Fridlund, B. (2000) Psychiatric nurses' conceptions of how group supervision in nursing care influences their professional competence. *Journal of Nursing Management*, 8 (3), pp. 175–185.

Arvidsson, B., Lofgren, H., Fridlund, B. (2001) Psychiatric nurses' conceptions of how a group supervision programme in nursing care influences their professional competence: a 4-year follow-up study. *Journal of Nursing Management*, 9 (3), pp. 161–171.

Ashmore, R. (1999) Heron's intervention framework: an introduction and critique. *Mental Health Nursing*, 19 (1), pp. 24–27.

Ashmore, R., Banks, D. (1997) Student nurses' perceptions of their interpersonal skills: a re-examination of Burnard and Morrison's findings. *International Journal of Nursing Studies*, 34 (5), pp. 335–345.

Ashmore, R., Carver, N. (2000) Clinical supervision in mental health nursing courses. *British Journal of Nursing*, 9 (3), pp. 171–176.

Austin, L., Luker, K., Caress, A., Hallet, C. (2000) Palliative care: community nurses' perceptions of quality. *Quality in Health Care*, 9 (3), pp. 151–158.

Babbie, E. (1979) *The Practice of Social Research*, Wadsworth Publishing, Belmot, CA.

Bainbridge, D., Butterworth, C., Mills, C. (2001) Clinical supervision. *Occupational Health*, 53 (3), pp. 16–17.

Barber, P., Norman, I. (1987) Skills in supervision. *Nursing Times*, 87 (1), pp. 56–57.

Barber, P., Norman, I. (1989) Preparing teachers for the performance and evaluation of gaming simulation in experiential learning climates. *Journal of Advanced Nursing*, 14 (1), pp. 146–151.

Barker, P.J. (1996) Interview, in *The Research Process in Nursing*, 3rd edn, (ed. D.F.S. Cormack), Blackwell Science, London, pp. 226–235.

Barker, P.J. (1999) *The Philosophy and Practice of Psychiatric Nursing*, Churchill Livingstone, Edinburgh.

Bartle, J. (2000) Clinical supervision: its place within the quality agenda. *Nursing Management*, 7 (5), pp. 30–33.

Basch, C.E. (1987) Focus group interview: an underutilised research technique for improving theory and practice in health education. *Health Education Journal*, 14 (4), pp. 411–448.

Bassett, C. (1999) Clinical supervision in perioperative practice. *British Journal of Theatre Nursing*, 9 (7), pp. 297–302.

Bassett, C. (2000) *Clinical Supervision: A Guide for Implementation*, Nursing Times Books, London.

Begat, I.B.E., Severinsson, E.I., Berggren, I.B. (1997) Implementation of clinical supervision in a medical department: nurses' views of the effects. *Journal of Clinical Nursing*, 6 (5), pp. 389–394.

Begley, C.M. (1996) Using triangulation in nursing research. *Journal of Advanced Nursing*, 24 (1), pp. 122–128.

Belcher, J.R., Fish, L.J.B. (1985) Hildegard Peplau, in *Nursing Theories: The Base For Professional Nursing Practice*, 2nd edn, (ed. J.B. George), Prentice Hall International, New Jersey, pp. 50–68.

Benfer, B.A. (1979) Clinical supervision as a support system for the care-giver. *Perspective in Psychiatric Care*, 17 (1), pp. 13–17.

Benner, P. (1984) *From Novice to Expert: Excellence and Power in Clinical Nursing Practice*, Addison-Wesley, London.

Berg, A., Hansson, U.W., Hallberg, I.R. (1994) Nurses' creativity, tedium and burnout during one year of clinical supervision and implementation of individualised patient nursing care: comparisons between a ward for severely demented patients and a similar control ward. *Journal of Advanced Nursing*, 20 (4), pp. 742–749.

Berg, B.L. (1989) *Qualitative Research Methods for the Social Sciences*, Allyn & Bacon, New York.

Bernard, J.M., Goodyear, R.K. (1998) *Fundamentals of Clinical Supervision*, Allyn & Bacon, London.

Billington, D., Hallinan, C., Robinson, A. (2005) Propelling towards professional supervision. *Occupational Health*, 57 (2), pp. 24–28.

Bishop, V. (1994) Clinical supervision for an accountable profession. *Nursing Times*, 90 (39), pp. 35–37.

Bishop, V. (1998a) *Clinical Supervision in Practice: Some Questions, Answers and Guidelines*, MacMillan Press, London.

Bishop, V. (1998b) Clinical supervision: what is going on? Results of a questionnaire. *Nursing Times Research*, 3 (2), pp. 141–150.

Blake, R.R., Mouton, J.S. (1976) *Consultation*, Addison-Wesley, London.

Blumberg, A. (1970) A system for analyzing supervisor–teacher interactions, in *Mirrors for Behaviour*, (eds A. Simon, G. Boyer), Research for Better Schools, Philadelphia, p. 3.

Bond, M., Holland, S. (1998) *Skills of Clinical Supervision: A Practical Guide for Supervisees, Clinical Supervisors and Managers*, Open University Press, Buckingham.

Bowles, N., Young, C. (1998) Clinical supervision: partnerships for sound practice. *Nursing Times Learning Curve*, 2 (10), pp. 7–8.

Bowles, N., Young, C. (1999) An evaluative study of clinical supervision based on Proctor's three function interactive model. *Journal of Advanced Nursing*, 30 (4), pp. 958–964.

Boyle, A., Grap, M.J., Younger, J., Thornby, D. (1991) Personal hardiness: ways of coping, social support and burnout in critical care. *Journal of Advanced Nursing*, 16 (7), pp. 850–857.

Bray, J. (1999) An ethnographic study of psychiatric nursing. *Journal of Psychiatric and Mental Health Nursing*, 6 (4), pp. 297–305.

Breeze, J.A., Repper, J. (1998) Struggling for control: the care experiences of 'difficult' patients in mental health services. *Journal of Advanced Nursing*, 28 (6), pp. 1301–1311.

Brenner, M., Brown, J., Canter, D. (1985) *The Research Interview: Uses and Approaches*, Academic Press, London.

Brink, P.J., Wood, M.J. (1994) *Basic Steps in Planning Nursing Research: From Question to Proposal*, Jones and Bartlett, London.

Brocklehurst, N. (1998) Clinical supervision in nursing homes. *Nursing Times*, 93 (12), pp. 39–40.

Brooker, C., White, E. (1997) *The Fourth Quinquennial National Community Mental Health Nursing Census of Northern Ireland*, University of Sheffield and Keele University, Sheffield.

Bulmer, C. (1997) Supervision: how it works. *Nursing Times*, 93 (48), pp. 53–54.

Burden, B. (1998) Illuminative evaluation. *Educational and Child Psychology*, 15 (3), pp. 15–23.

Burnard, P. (1985) *Learning Human Skills: A Guide for Nurses*, Heinemann, London.

Burnard, P. (1991) A method of analysing interview transcripts in qualitative research. *Nurse Education Today*, 11 (4), pp. 461–466.

Burnard, P. (2002) *Learning Human Skills: An Experiential and Reflective Guide for Nurses and Health Care Professionals*, 4th edn, Butterworth-Heinemann, Oxford.

Burnard, P., Edwards, D., Fothergill, A. *et al.* (2000) Community mental health nurses in Wales: self-reported stressors and coping strategies. *Journal of Psychiatric and Mental Health Nursing*, 7 (6), pp. 523–528.

Burnard, P., Morrison, P. (1988) Nurses' perceptions of their interpersonal skills: a descriptive study using Six Category Intervention Analysis. *Nurse Education Today*, 8 (5), pp. 266–272.

Burnard, P., Morrison, P. (1991) Nurses' interpersonal skills: a study of nurses' perceptions. *Nurse Education Today*, 11 (1), pp. 24–29.

Burns, M.E. (1958) *The Historical Development of the Process of Casework Supervision as seen in the Professional Literature of Social Work*, Department of Social Work, University of Chicago, Chicago.

Burrow, S. (1995) Supervision: clinical development or management control? *British Journal of Nursing*, 4 (15), pp. 879–882.

Butcher, K. (1995) Taking notes. *Nursing Times*, 91 (1), p. 33.

Butterworth, T. (1996) Primary attempts at research-based evaluation of clinical supervision. *Nursing Times Research*, 1 (2), pp. 96–101.

Butterworth, T., Carson, J., Jeacock, J. *et al.* (1999) Stress, coping, burnout and job satisfaction in British nurses: findings from the clinical supervision evaluation project. *Stress Medicine*, 15 (1), pp. 27–33.

Butterworth, T., Carson, J., White, E. *et al.* (1997) *It Is Good To Talk: An Evaluation Study in England and Scotland*, University of Manchester, Manchester.

Butterworth, T., Faugier, J. (1992) *Clinical Supervision and Mentorship in Nursing*, Chapman and Hall, London.

Butterworth, T., Faugier, J., Burnard, P. (1998a) *Clinical Supervision and Mentorship in Nursing*, 2nd edn, Nelson Thornes Ltd, Cheltenham.

Butterworth, T., White, E., Carson, J. *et al.* (1998b) Developing and evaluating clinical supervision in the United Kingdom. *EDTNA / ERCA Journal*, 24 (1), pp. 2–8, 12.

Butterworth, T., Woods D. (1999) *Clinical Governance and Clinical Supervision: Working together to ensure safe and accountable practice. A briefing paper*, University of Manchester, Manchester.

Campbell, D.T., Fiske, D.W. (1959) Convergent and discriminant validity by the multi-trait, multi-method matrix. *Psychological Bulletin*, 56 (1), pp. 81–105.

Carifio, M.S., Hess, A.K. (1987) Who is the ideal supervisor? *Professional Psychology: Research and Practice*, 18 (3), pp. 244–250.

Carthy, J. (1994) Bandwagons roll. *Nursing Standard*, 8 (38), pp. 48–49.

Cerinus, M. (2003) *An Exploration of the Change Required to Support the Introduction of Clinical Supervision*, Glasgow Caledonian University, Glasgow. PhD dissertation.

Chambers, M. (1988) Curriculum evaluation: An approach towards appraising a post-basic psychiatric nursing course. *Journal of Advanced Nursing*, 13 (3), pp. 330–340.

Chambers, M. (1990) Psychiatric and mental health nursing: learning in the clinical environment, in *Psychiatric and Mental Health Nursing: Theory and Practice*, (eds W. Reynolds, D. Cormack), Chapman and Hall, London, pp. 396–433.

Chambers, M., Cutcliffe, J. (2001) The dynamics and processes of 'ending' in clinical supervision. *British Journal of Nursing*, 10 (21), pp. 1403–1411.

Chambers, M., Long, A. (1995) Supportive clinical supervision: A crucible for personal and professional change. *Journal of Psychiatric and Mental Health Nursing*, 2 (5), pp. 311–316.

Cheater, F.M., Hale, C. (2001) An evaluation of a local clinical supervision scheme for practice nurses. *Journal of Clinical Nursing*, 10 (1), pp 119–131.

Chinn, P.L. (1986) *Nursing Research Methodology: Issues and Implementation*, Aspen Publications, Royal Turnbridge Wells.

Chorley, A., Kitney, J. (2000) Practice makes perfect. *Occupational Health*, 52 (5), p. 28.

Christman, N.J., Johnson, J.E. (1981) Ethics: human subjects in research, in *Research Methodology and its Application to Nursing*, (ed. Y.M. Williamson), John Wiley & Sons, New York, pp. 25–39.

Clamp, C. (1980) Learning through incidents. *Nursing Times*, 76 (40), pp. 1755–1758.

Claveirole, A., Mathers, M. (2003) Peer supervision: an experimental scheme for nurse lecturers. *Nurse Education Today*, 23 (1), pp. 51–57.

Clifton, E. (2002) Implementing clinical supervision. *Nursing Times*, 98 (9), pp. 36–37.

Clothier, C., MacDonald, C.A., Shaw, D.A. (1994) *The Allitt Inquiry: Independent Inquiry relating to the Deaths and Injuries on the Children's Ward at Grantham and Kesteven General Hospital during the period February to April 1991*, HMSO, London.

Clough, A. (2001) Clinical leadership: turning thought into action. *Primary Health Care*, 11 (4), pp. 39–41.

Coffey, M., Coleman, M. (2001) The relationship between support and stress in forensic mental health nursing. *Journal of Advanced Nursing*, 34 (3), pp. 397–407.

Cole, A. (2002) Someone to watch over you. *Nursing Times*, 98 (23), pp. 22–25.

Coleman, M., Rafferty, M. (1995) Using workshops to implement clinical supervision. *Nursing Standard*, 9 (1), pp. 30–34.

Community Psychiatric Nurses Association (1985) *The Clinical Nursing Responsibilities of the Community Psychiatric Nurse*, CPNA, Bristol.

Consedine, M. (2000) Developing abilities: the future of clinical supervision? *Journal of Psychiatric and Mental Health Nursing*, 7 (5), pp. 467–474.

Conway, J.E. (1998) Evolution of the species 'expert nurse': an examination of the practical knowledge held by nurses. *Journal of Clinical Nursing*, 7 (1), pp. 75–82.

Cook, R. (1996) Clinical supervision: a talking shop. Practice Nursing, 7 (15), pp. 12–13.

Coombes, R. (1997) Clinical supervision brings little gain. *Nursing Times*, 93 (23), p. 7.

Cormack, D. (1976) *Psychiatric Nursing Observed: A Descriptive Study of the Work of the Charge Nurse in Acute Admission Wards of Psychiatric Hospitals*, RCN, London.

Cormack, D.E.F. (1983) *Psychiatric Nursing Described*, Churchill Livingstone, London.

Corner, C. (1991) In search of more complete answers to research questions. Quantitative versus qualitative research methods: is there a way forward? *Journal of Advanced Nursing*, 16 (6), pp. 718–727.

Cotton, A. (2001) Clinical supervision UK style: good for nurses and nursing? *Contemporary Nurse*, 11 (1), pp. 60–70.

Cottrell, S. (2001) Occupational stress and job satisfaction in mental health nursing: focused interventions through evidence-based assessment. *Journal of Psychiatric and Mental Health Nursing*, 8 (2), pp. 157–164.

Cowley, S. (1995) Professional development and change in a learning organisation. *Journal of Advanced Nursing*, 21 (5), pp. 965–974.

Critchley, D.L. (1987) Clinical supervision as a learning tool for the therapist in milieu settings. *Journal of Psychosocial Nursing*, 25 (8), pp. 18–22.

Crotty, M. (1990) The perceptions of students and teachers regarding the introductory module of an enrolled nurse conversion course. *Nurse Education Today*, 10 (5), pp. 366–379.

Cutcliffe, J. (2000a) Should line managers be supervisors? *British Journal of Nursing*, 9 (22), p. 2268.

Cutcliffe, J. (2000b) To record or not to record: documentation in clinical supervision. *British Journal of Nursing*, 9 (6), pp. 350–355.

Cutcliffe, J., Burns, J. (1998) Personal, professional and practice development: clinical supervision. *British Journal of Nursing*, 7 (21), pp. 1318–1321.

Cutcliffe, J., Butterworth, T., Proctor, B. (2001) *Fundamental Themes in Clinical Supervision*, Routledge, London.

Cutcliffe, J., Epling, M. (1997) An exploration of the use of John Heron's confronting interventions in clinical supervision: case studies from practice. *Psychiatric Care*, 4 (4), pp. 174–180.

Cutcliffe, J., McKenna, H.P. (1999) Establishing the credibility of qualitative research findings: the plot thickens. *Journal of Advanced Nursing*, 30 (2), pp. 374–380.

Cutcliffe, J., Proctor, B. (1998) An alternative training approach to clinical supervision: 1. *British Journal of Nursing*, 7 (5), pp. 280–285.

Dachelet, C.Z., Wemett, M.F., Garling, E.J. *et al.* (1981) The critical incident technique applied to the evaluation of the clinical practicum setting. *Journal of Nursing Education*, 20 (8), pp. 15–31.

Darley, G. (2001) Demystifying supervision. *Nursing Management*, 7 (10), pp. 18–21.

Darling, L. (1984) What do nurses want in a mentor? *Journal of Nursing Administration*, 14 (10), pp. 42–44.

Dartington, A. (1993) Where angels fear to tread: idealism, despondency, and inhibition in thought in hospital nursing. *Winnicott Studies*, 7 (1), pp. 21–41.

Davidson, J. (1998) Snapshots from Scotland, in *Clinical Supervision in Practice: Some questions, answers and guidelines*, (ed. V. Bishop), MacMillan Press, London, pp. 24–33.

Davies, P. (1993) Value yourself. *Nursing Times*, 89 (4), p. 52.

Davy, J. (2002) Discursive reflections on a research agenda for clinical supervision. *Psychology and Psychotherapy: Theory, Research and Practice*, 75 (2), pp. 221–238.

De Raeve, L. (1998) Maintaining integrity through clinical supervision. *Nursing Ethics*, 5 (6), pp. 486–496.

De Shazer, S. (1985) *Keys to Solutions in Brief Therapy*, Norton & Company, New York.

Denzin, N.K. (1970) *The Research Act in Society: A Theoretical Introduction to Sociological Methods*, Butterworth, London.

Denzin, N.K. (1989) *The Research Act: A Theoretical Introduction to Sociological Methods*, 3rd edn, Prentice Hall, New Jersey.

Department of Health (1993) *A Vision for the Future: The Nursing, Midwifery and Health Visiting Contribution to Health and Health Care*, HMSO, London.

Department of Health (1994a) *CNO Letter 94 (5) Clinical supervision for the nursing and health visiting professions*, HMSO, London.

Department of Health (1994b) *Working in Partnership: A Collaborative Approach to Care. Report of the Mental Health Nursing Review Team*, HMSO, London.

Department of Health (1999) *Making a Difference: Strengthening the Nursing, Midwifery and Health Visiting Contribution to Health and Health Care*, HMSO, London.

Devitt, P. (1998) *A grounded theory investigation into the nature of the supervisory relationship and the labour of supervision through the eyes of the supervisor*. Department of Nursing, University of Manchester, Manchester. MSc dissertation.

Dewar, B.J., Walker, E. (1999) Experiential learning: issues for supervision. *Journal of Advanced Nursing*, 30 (6), pp. 1459–1467.

Dixon, A., Bramwell, R. (2001) Neonatal nurses' attitudes to clinical supervision: results of a survey. *Journal of Neonatal Nursing*, 7 (1), pp. 20–24.

Docherty, B. (2000) Negotiating management and staff needs. *Nursing Times*, 96 (14), pp. 45–48.

Doehrmann, M.J. (1976) Parallel processes in supervision and psychotherapy. *Bulletin of the Menninger Clinic*, 40 (1), pp. 3–104.

Draper, B., Koukos, C., Fletcher, P. *et al.* (1999) Evaluating an initiative: clinical supervision in a community health trust. *British Journal of Community Nursing*, 4 (10), pp. 525–530.

Driscoll, J. (1999) Getting the most from clinical supervision. Part one: the supervisee. *Mental Health Practice*, 2 (6), pp. 28–35.

Driscoll, J. (2000a) *Practising Clinical Supervision: A Reflective Approach*, Bailliere Tindall, London.

Driscoll, J. (2000b) Clinical supervision: a radical approach. *Mental Health Practice*, 3 (8), pp. 8–10.

Drummond, J.S. (1990) The work style of students of mental health nursing undertaking the Project 2000 scheme of training: a logical analysis. *Journal of Advanced Nursing*, 15 (8), pp. 977–984.

Duarri, W., Kendrick, K. (1999) Implementing clinical supervision. *Professional Nurse*, 14 (12), pp. 849–852.

Dudley, M., Butterworth, T. (1994) The cost and some benefits of clinical supervision: an initial exploration. *International Journal of Psychiatric Nursing Research*, 1 (2), pp. 34–40.

Smith, D. (2001) Introducing clinical supervision: the pitfalls and problems. *British Journal of Perioperative Nursing*, 11 (10), pp. 436–441.

Smith, L. (1992) Ethical issues in interviewing. *Journal of Advanced Nursing*, 17 (1), pp. 98–103.

Smith, P., Masterson, A., Lask, S. (1995) Health and the curriculum: an illuminative evaluation–part one: Methodology. *Nurse Education Today*, 15 (4), pp. 245–249.

Spence, C., Cantrell, J., Christie, J., Samet, W. (2002) A collaborative approach to the implementation of clinical supervision. *Journal of Nursing Management*, 10 (2), pp. 65–74.

Stevenson, C., Jackson, B. (2000) Egalitarian consultation meetings: an alternative to received wisdom about clinical supervision in psychiatric nursing practice. *Journal of Psychiatric and Mental Health Nursing*, 7 (6), pp. 491–504.

Streubert, H.J., Carpenter, D.R. (1999) *Qualitative Research in Nursing: Advancing the Humanistic Imperative*, Lippincott, New York.

Styles, J., Gibson, T. (1999) Is clinical supervision an option for practice nurses? *Practice Nursing*, 10 (11), pp. 10–14.

Sullivan, P. (1998) Therapeutic interaction and mental health nursing. *Nursing Standard*, 12 (45), pp. 39–42.

Swain, G. (1995) *Clinical Supervision: The Principles and Process*, Health Visitors Association, London.

Tapp, D.M., Wright, L.M. (1996) Live supervision and family systems nursing: postmodern influences and dilemmas. *Journal of Psychiatric and Mental Health Nursing*, 3 (4), pp. 225–233.

Teasdale, K. (2000) Practical approaches to clinical supervision. *Professional Nurse*, 15 (9), pp. 579–582.

Teasdale, K., Brocklehurst, N., Thom, N. (2001) Clinical supervision and support for nurses: an evaluation study. *Journal of Advanced Nursing*, 33 (2), pp. 216–224.

Teasdale, K., Thom, N., Brocklehurst, N. (1998) *The Value of Clinical Supervision in Nursing: A Research Study Commissioned by the NHS Executive in Trent*, South Lincolnshire Training and Development Partnership, Boston.

Temple, S., Bowers, W.A. (1998) Supervising cognitive therapists from diverse fields. *Journal of Cognitive Psychotherapy: An International Quarterly*, 12 (2), pp. 139–151.

Termini, M., Hauser, M.J. (1973) The process of the supervisory relationship. *Perspectives in Psychiatric Care*, 11 (3), pp. 121–125.

Thompson, C. (2003) Clinical experience as evidence in evidence-based practice. *Journal of Advanced Nursing*, 43 (3), pp. 230–237.

Timpson, J. (1996) Clinical supervision: a plea for 'pit head time' in cancer nursing. *European Journal of Cancer Nursing*, 5 (1), pp. 43–52.

Tingle, J. (1995) Clinical supervision is an effective risk management tool. *British Journal of Nursing*, 4 (14), pp. 794–795.

Todd, G., Freshwater, D. (1999) Reflective practice and guided discovery: clinical supervision. *British Journal of Nursing*, 8 (20), pp. 1383–1389.

Towell, D. (1975) *Understanding Psychiatric Nursing: A Sociological Study of Modern Psychiatric Nursing Practice*, RCN, London.

Trainor, M.A. (1978) A helping model for clinical supervision. *Supervisor Nurse*, 9 (1), pp. 30–36.

Travelbee, J. (1971) *Interpersonal Aspects of Nursing*, F.A. Davis, Philadelphia.

Tripp, D. (1993) *Critical Incidents in Teaching*, Routledge, London.

United Kingdom Central Council for Nursing, Midwifery and Health Visiting (1986) *A New Preparation for Practice*, UKCC, London.

United Kingdom Central Council For Nursing, Midwifery and Health Visiting (1990) *Discussion Paper on Post-Registration Education and Practice*, UKCC, London.

United Kingdom Central Council for Nursing, Midwifery and Health Visiting (1995) *Position Statement on Clinical Supervision for Nursing and Health Visiting*, UKCC, London.

United Kingdom Central Council for Nursing, Midwifery and Health Visiting (1996) *Position Statement on Clinical Supervision for Nursing and Health Visiting*, UKCC, London.

United Kingdom Central Council for Nursing, Midwifery and Health Visiting (2001) *Supporting Nurses, Midwives and Health Visitors Through Lifelong Learning*, UKCC, London.

Van Ooijen, E. (1994) Whipping up a storm . . . use clinical supervision in a punitive, controlling way? *Nursing Standard*, 9 (8), p. 48.

Van Ooijen, E. (2000) *Clinical Supervision: A Practical Guide*, Churchill Livingstone, London.

Veeramah, V. (2002) The benefits of using clinical supervision. *Mental Health Nursing*, 22 (1), pp. 18–23.

Veitch, L., May, N., McIntosh, J. (1997) The practice-based context of educational innovation: nurse and midwife preparation in Scotland. *Journal of Advanced Nursing*, 25 (1), pp. 191–198.

Walker, R., Clark, J.J. (1999) Heading off boundary problems: clinical supervision as risk management. *Psychiatric Services*, 50 (11), pp. 1435–1439.

Walsh, K., Nicholson, J., Keough, C. *et al.* (2003) Development of a group model of clinical supervision to meet the needs of a community mental health nursing team. *International Journal of Nursing Practice*, 9 (1), pp. 33–39.

Walsh, M. (1991) *Models in Clinical Nursing: The Way Forward*, Bailliere Tindall, London.

Ward, M., Cutcliffe, J., Gournay, K. (2000) *The Nursing, Midwifery and Health Visiting Contribution to the Continuing Care of People with Mental Health Problems: A Review and UKCC Action Plan*, UKCC, London.

Waterworth, S., Pilliteri, L., Swift, F. (1997) Clinical supervision: empowerment in practice. *Nursing Management*, 3 (9), pp. 14–16.

Watkins, C.E. (1990) The separation-individuation process in psychotherapy supervision. *Psychotherapy*, 27 (2), pp. 202–209.

Watkins, C.E. (1995) Psychotherapy supervision in the 1990's: some observations and reflections. *American Journal of Psychotherapy*, 49 (4), pp. 568–581.

White, E., Butterworth, T., Bishop, V. *et al.* (1998) Clinical supervision: insider reports of a private world. *Journal of Advanced Nursing*, 28 (1), pp. 185–192.

Whittaker, J., Ball, C. (2000) Discharge from intensive care: a view from the ward. *Intensive and Critical Care Nursing*, 16 (3), pp. 135–143.

Whyte, R., Watson, H. (1998) Developing research methods in qualitative research: using a radio microphone in a pilot study. *Nurse Researcher*, 6 (1), pp. 60–71.

Wikberg, A., Jansson, L., Lithner, F. (2000) Women's experience of suffering repeated severe attacks of acute intermittent porphyria. *Journal of Advanced Nursing*, 32 (6), pp. 1348–1355.

Wilkin, P. (1988) Someone to watch over me. *Nursing Times*, 84 (33), pp. 33–34.

The Yearbook of
OBSTETRICS
and
GYNAECOLOGY

Volume 10

Edited by
David Sturdee, Karl Oláh, David Purdie and
Declan Keane

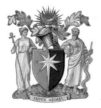

RCOG Press

Published by the **RCOG Press** at the
Royal College of Obstetricians and Gynaecologists
27 Sussex Place, Regent's Park
London NW1 4RG
Registered Charity No. 213280

RCOG Press Editor: Sophie Leighton
Cover designed by Geoffrey Wadsley
Typeset by FiSH Books, London